HEALING
WITH
SHUNGITE

HEALING
WITH
SHUNGITE

The Complete Guide for Protecting, Detoxing, and Purifying Your Mind, Body, and Soul

Jessica Mahler

Published in the US by:
ULYSSES PRESS
PO Box 3440
Berkeley, CA 94703
www.ulyssespress.com

ISBN: 978-1-64604-091-9
Library of Congress Control Number: 2020936175

Printed in Canada by Marquis Book Printing
10 9 8 7 6 5 4 3 2 1

Acquisitions editor: Casie Vogel
Managing editor: Claire Chun
Project editor: Tyanni Niles
Editors: Scott Calamar, Renee Rutledge
Proofreader: Anne Healey
Front cover design: Rebecca Lown
Cover art: hands © ex_atist/shutterstock.com
Interior design: what!design @ whatweb.com
Layout: Jake Flaherty

For anyone who's ever been told they're too sensitive

Contents

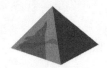

Preface: My Journey with Shungite

Shungite first came into my life in 2016. I was covering a vegan food festival in Miami where, sandwiched between vendors offering samples of organic vegan cupcakes and sustainably sourced coffee, I found a table covered in black crystals. I've always had a fascination with crystals, dating back to grade school, when I would blow several weeks of saved allowance at the Natural History Museum gift shop on pretty pebbles with healing abilities that meant nothing to me at the time; I was just overcome with a deep knowing that I had to have them. Fast-forward three decades, and here I am, still spending my hard-earned money on crystals and minerals with healing abilities to assist my life and the lives of those I work with one-on-one.

When I met this particular vendor, she only spoke of shungite's ability to protect against electromagnetic fields (EMFs) and calm anxiety. As someone who suffered from crippling anxiety for the first twenty-five years of my life, my ears perked up at the notion that this crystal I had never heard of could help me keep my tendency to worry and overthink in check.

I had been feeling a bit like a fish out of water at the festival; this was the first time I had ever been flown somewhere for a story, and I was extremely nervous—not because I was traveling by myself, but because of the immense pressure I placed on myself to make sure I was at as many events as possible to find the best story angles and get the best interviews. I have always been particularly sensitive. But when I held the shungite in my hand that day, a sense of calm washed over me. In a warehouse filled with the din of conversation and movement that had previously made me feel uneasy and on edge, I suddenly felt—at peace. With everything. I'd like two, please.

This book was written entirely during the COVID-19 pandemic. I had been traveling around the world for two months for various work and personal reasons. At the time of my travels, the coronavirus scare hadn't hit the locations I had been touring, so returning home March 2020 to the US in panic mode felt like I had landed in a parallel universe. The world seemed to have completely shut down, and with it, my career. Not only did I have classes, workshops, and trainings to cancel, but I also had two retreats to reschedule. Losing out on the income I thought I was coming home to, I could have freaked out. But meditating with shungite daily and placing it all around my home kept me not only sane but also hopeful for what was to come. Where the old me might have been hyperventilating, present me took many long, deep breaths, grabbed my shungite, and stayed calm.

My relationship with anxiety definitely took some time to understand. I had suffered from insomnia since I was born and wouldn't get regular full nights of sleep until my late twenties. I first looked to yoga twenty years ago thanks to my mother, who believed starting a yoga practice would help my thoughts from racing at night so that I could sleep more soundly. My interest in yoga led me to more esoteric practices of Reiki and breathwork. And while all these tools have been positive influences that helped me to uncover the stories from my life that have contributed to my nervous proclivities, it wasn't until I began to intentionally work with shungite that I noticed a significant difference in my overall mindset and energy.

Which isn't to say that helping to ease anxiety is all that shungite is capable of. On the contrary, I've found that it can actually help in myriad ways in various areas of our lives. Understanding the effects of shungite's energy helped me recognize how our modern-day ailments are associated with both our surroundings and our life experiences. This helped me to connect the dots between the physical realm and the energy realm. My hope is that this book helps you to do the same.

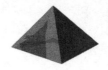

Introduction

The popularity of healing crystals wasn't born out of the New Age movement that exploded in Western culture in the 1970s. The flower power counterculture that erupted in the late '60s and early '70s promoted peace, equality, nonviolence, and love in opposition to a disappointing, corrupt US government. At the time, the US was engulfed with Vietnam in one of the most unpopular military conflicts on record. With the end of the war, the peace-and-love resistance eventually gave way to a new era touting practices in search of a deeper meaning to life. People began to turn their awareness inward.

The term *New Age* is deceiving; this movement didn't actually promote anything "new." As therapy became more popular and gained acceptance as a means to heal trauma and post-traumatic stress disorder (PTSD), people began to look to a variety of ancient cultures in their search for personal transformation. It was at this time that interest in Buddhism, yoga, meditation, acupuncture, natural food diets, astrology, and other spiritual disciplines exploded onto the scene as ways to assist planetary healing and societal revolution.

Crystal healing was one of these alternative modalities for those seeking the transformation and wholeness that they purportedly were capable of. Thought to be great reservoirs of energy that could be released for personal benefit, crystals became the most popular items available at the metaphysical shops that began popping up in the '80s, and they continue to be best sellers today.

We've come a long way since the Sumerians and ancient Egyptians first began looking to stones for protection. But their findings and beliefs in their work with crystals have followed us through time, embedding themselves in our DNA. Because they looked to stones for help, so did the civilizations that followed, riding generation after generation.

Our modern-day problems may be different, but the antidote remains the same: crystals.

Crystals have an air about them that makes them seem unexplainable, magical even. The word *crystal* is actually derived from the Greek word for *ice*: *krystallos*. The Greeks believed that, since the unique look, shape, and luster of crystals so closely resembled ice, these minerals were actually frozen water formed so deep in a body of water that they could never be unfrozen. They were awestruck by the light-reflecting qualities of this "ice."

We have long believed crystals to restore and enhance physical, mental, emotional, and spiritual equilibrium. There was no research to back the claims of ancient civilizations, just experience and belief. The Greeks, in fact, learned how to work with crystals from the Persians after winning the Persian War. And though we've relied heavily on the ideas and beliefs about how to work with crystals that have been passed down generational lines, there is a science to it as well. This book attempts to take an in-depth look at how the planet's formation plays an integral role in the energies of these mysterious pieces of earth to help us understand how one mineral in particular—shungite—is capable of so much.

The word *crystal* is used liberally today. Not all healing stones look like the "ice" the Greeks were mesmerized by, but we've come to group all stones we use for healing as crystals. This is probably because the word *crystal* has an enchanting connotation to it: the idea of a rock having invisible characteristics that help facilitate healing can seem a bit fantastical to nonbelievers. While it isn't completely wrong to use the term so enthusiastically, it's not 100 percent accurate 100 percent of the time. Science has taught us a lot about our friends from the earth: what classifies a crystal as a crystal isn't its sheen or gleaming qualities but its internal structure, or crystal lattice. Shungite is classified as a mineral, which by definition is considered a crystal, but it's a bit deeper than that. We'll talk more about this distinction in Chapter One. I'll be using the words *crystal* and *mineral* interchangeably in this book.

To understand why shungite has gotten such a buzz around it, we have to look at the problems that plague today's society. Up until five hundred years ago, civilization was based on theology. Deeply entrenched in polytheistic and monotheistic beliefs, humans feared the gods they worshipped, unable to fathom a world where man could surpass human limitations, as described in religious texts. For much of our existence, it was believed that to do so would only end in disappointment or disaster. The dawning of the Renaissance led us out of the Middle Ages and into the modern age. With new ways of thinking, humans began to question their potential and what was possible. Our earlier ancestors took what they knew at face value, afraid to question the creations of the gods. But with the Renaissance, which literally means the revival or renewed interest in something, we began to understand that there was so much we didn't know. So we started to ask questions.

As scientific discoveries helped us solve one problem after another, we went from feeling limited in what we were capable of to believing we, like the gods, were limit*less*. As our technology and understanding of the human body improved, suddenly, being sick wasn't a death sentence; outsmarting death would become our obsession, and it continues to propel tests, studies, and technology to see if perhaps one day we might be able to dodge the inevitable.

The Renaissance was our launchpad into the future, into the unknown. Electricity was discovered less than three hundred years ago, and we have done so much with it since. First it allowed us to communicate with friends and loved ones in different parts of the country and, eventually, the world; then we learned how to wire our homes in order to have light whenever we needed it. It helped us update our iceboxes in order to keep our food fresh for longer. It made doing laundry less time-consuming; it took us to the moon. As we've become emboldened to ask, "What if?" more frequently, so, too, has our technology improved. But it all comes at a price.

We couldn't know that, while we were attempting to make our lives easier, we were also creating new problems, new byproducts that would have lasting, palpable effects.

This book also attempts to look at how our technological advancements are affecting the body from the inside out and, looking back on our fascination with crystals, how shungite is the antidote for these modern dilemmas. Together we will investigate the energy of the human body, learn how rocks and crystals are formed, and discover how their birth stories affect their power and effectiveness in helping the human energy field. We'll take a look at how EMFs work and the effects of our exposure to them, why anxiety is at an all-time high and how it shows up in the human body, and the relationship between EMF exposure and anxiety. We'll journey through the chakras to understand how our experiences and traumas affect us, and we'll see how anxiety manifests differently in everyone and can be triggered by different things. And you'll learn ways to work with shungite to help protect yourself from EMFs, calm anxiety, and help you heal.

To understand why and how crystals work, and why you're here to learn more about our friend shungite, first we have to travel back in time to look at how crystals are formed and visit with the cultures that passed down crystal healing practices that continue to inspire and resonate with us today.

CHAPTER 1

What Is Shungite?

All rocks have a creation story.

Some have been melted, some burned. Some were created under intense pressure, some hold and retain moisture, some coagulated from concentrated drips (think stalactites and stalagmites, those icicle-looking rocks that grow toward one another on the roofs and floors of caves, respectively). They differ in density, weight, and luster. Some are solid in color, others are variegated. Some cannot be cut and only exist as how they were formed, while others crumble to the touch if you apply too much pressure.

The story of how a rock or crystal is formed directly affects the power or energy that it gives off or attracts.

Just as astrologers look to the exact time and place of your birth to understand your personality, strengths, weaknesses, and life purpose—the core tenet of astrology is that the map of the sky at the time you were born plays a significant role in who you came here to be and all the highs and lows you may face in this lifetime—the time and location crystals were formed affect their properties and the energy they absorb, enhance, attract, or emit.

DEFINITION OF SHUNGITE

Shungite is classified as an amorphous (meaning it cooled extremely fast) metamorphic mineral. It started off as a different type of rock altogether, but extreme heat and pressure within the earth's crust transformed its mineral makeup to become what we know as shungite today. Geologists believe that shungite first formed during the Paleoproterozoic Era, the longest era in the earth's geological formation, 2.5 to 1.6 billion years ago. It was first discovered in seventeenth-century Russia in Karelia, near Shun'ga village, where shungite's name is derived from. Shungite is only found naturally in northwest Russia, in the upper Zaonezhskaya Formation, just northeast of St. Petersburg.[1]

THE DIFFERENT TYPES OF SHUNGITE

There are three types of shungite.

TYPE I (ELITE SHUNGITE)

- Referred to as "silver shungite"

- Black in color, with a silvery shine

---

1   V. A. Melezhik et al. "Karelian Shungite—An Indication of 2.0-Ga-Old Metamorphosed Oil-Shale and Generation of Petroleum: Geology, Lithology and Geochemistry." *Earth-Science Reviews*, J47, nos. 1–2 (1999): 1—40, https://www .sciencedirect.com/science/article/abs/pii/S0012825299000276?via=ihub.

- Made up of 98 percent organic carbon, with trace amounts of nitrogen, sulfur, oxygen, and hydrogen
- Manually excavated
- Easily identified by its conchoidal fractures, smooth curves resembling a round snail shell, a physical attribute from cooling too quickly when it formed
- Sold in its natural shape
- Lightweight
- Extremely fragile
- Only available as a raw stone but sometimes sold as jewelry in its raw state
- The rarest shungite, making up only 1 percent of all shungite found in the world
- Due to its high carbon makeup, the most powerful and effective shungite
- Best used for water purification

TYPE II (PETROVSKY SHUNGITE)

- Grayish-black in color
- Made up of 64 percent organic carbon, 3.5 percent nitrogen, 3.5 percent oxygen, 6.7 percent hydrogen, and up to 3.3 percent ash
- Industrially mined

- Much sturdier than elite shungite

- Heavy in weight

- Easily shaped and polished, so it's used for jewelry and figurines

- Considered a transitional stone because it has all the healing properties of elite shungite and is almost as effective

TYPE III (REGULAR SHUNGITE)

- Black in color

- Made up of 30 to 50 percent organic carbon; up to 56 percent silicon dioxide; 4.2 percent water; 4 percent aluminum oxide; 2.5 percent iron oxide; 1.5 percent potassium oxide; 1.2 percent magnesium oxide; 1.2 percent sulfur; and trace amounts of calcium oxide, sodium oxide, or titanium oxide

- Sturdier than both Petrovsky and elite shungite

- In terms of weight, the heaviest type of shungite

- Easily shaped and polished, so commonly used for jewelry and figurines

- Commonly referred to as "shungite rock" since this type contains a much lower percentage of organic carbon than the other two

THE ELEMENTAL MAKEUP
OF SHUNGITE

It's shungite's high carbon makeup that gives the mineral certain catalytic abilities, making it especially good for electroconductivity and chemical resistance. This is the magic behind shungite's EMF-fighting capabilities. We'll discuss more about EMFs in Chapter Four.

But let's not get too far ahead of ourselves. To understand how shungite came to be, we have to start at the beginning.

All crystals start out as magma, that molten fluid found bubbling beneath the earth's crust. When magma makes its way above ground, it's considered lava, but the atmosphere is no longer hot enough to keep it in its liquid form. The cooling process of lava is what creates minerals or igneous rocks. All minerals start out as igneous rocks, but not all igneous rocks are the same. This is because magma contains many different mineral-forming elements.

Magma is the substance that created the surface of the earth. The movement or motion of magma has no ordered state. From a scientific point of view, it's believed that 4.5 billion years ago, planet Earth started out as a gigantic cloud of cosmic dust and gas. The force of gravity drew these particles together, eventually forming a blazingly hot liquid sphere. Over time, the temperature of the sphere decreased and its composition began to change. It's believed that around this time—about 3.5 billion years ago—the earth's magnetic field began to form. Eventually light matter and heavy matter separated—like oil and water—creating the different layers of the earth (core, mantle, crust), and the surface began to cool, creating a thin outer shell. This shell had many cracks in it; magma and steam forced their way through these cracks to create larger, thicker layers of rock that make up the earth's crust. With mantle flowing beneath the crust, large plates of rock (tectonic plates) began to shift: friction and collisions gave rise to mountains, volcanoes, and earthquakes, which shaped the surface of the earth.

From chaos, order was created.

Different substances commingle in magma, which informs us that the hot liquid is not a homogeneous substance; its makeup varies in different areas of the earth, which helps us understand why many different types of minerals are formed by magma. It's also the reason that distinctive minerals are only found in certain parts of the world.

Other factors also help determine the fate or distinction of a mineral. Once the mineral makes it to the earth's surface, outside forces like wind and water cause it to erode. Water in particular can completely dissolve certain mineral-forming elements, which then transforms the mineral's composition. If an igneous rock is weathered by the elements in a way that has changed its mineral makeup and/or if it's transported away from where it was created and deposited elsewhere via the wind or a body of water, then it's considered sedimentary rock.

And yet another type of rock is metamorphic—rock that has been transformed by extreme heat and pressure without becoming molten. The metamorphic process reorganizes the original structure of igneous or sedimentary rocks to create a stronger, more stable rock. This type of rock formation tends to occur deep within the earth's crust or at the site of colliding tectonic plates. When existing igneous and sedimentary rocks get folded back into the earth's crust, the increase in pressure causes them to restructure into new chemical compounds. Some substances from a rock's original makeup may quite literally get squeezed out; these compressed minerals accumulate to create new, more resistant minerals. You can actually see how a rock's composition has bent under pressure in the striations of color in metamorphic rock like tiger's-eye, lapis lazuli, and marble.

Time is also a factor. The longer the solidification process takes, the larger the crystal can grow; if the process is fast, the crystals are small. Sometimes the cooling happens at such a rapid pace that there is no time for crystalline structures to form, and the byproduct looks more like rock than the "ice" the Greeks referred to. It can take eons for a crystal to form, or mere seconds. Some are solidified via heat, others through freezing temperatures.

At its most basic, a crystal is a naturally occurring solid. Each type of crystal has its own precise atomic arrangement in a geometric crystal lattice that makes it unique to other classifications of crystals. Its organized structure is what provides its stability and the regularity of flow of any electromagnetic energies that pass through it. This internal structure defines a crystal.

A QUICK UNDERSTANDING OF TERMINOLOGY

Stone is the collective name for all solid, nonmetallic constituents of the earth's crust—save for ice and coal.

Rock is the natural aggregate of two or more minerals, which forms part of the surface of the earth and other similar planets, exposed on the surface or underlying the soil or oceans.

Crystal is a naturally occurring solid with a strict order of atoms, ions, and molecules positioned in exact distances and angles from one another in a geometric crystal lattice. This yields varying physical qualities; crystals have been shown to hold both heat and electricity, as well as to increase the frequency of light that passes through them.

Mineral is a naturally occurring, inorganic solid with a definitive chemical composition. By definition, all minerals must have a crystal structure; therefore, all minerals are crystals. This is shungite's classification.

While many different types of crystals may be formed out of the same mineral or combination of minerals, each type crystallizes in its own unique way. The same type of crystal may have several different colors or external forms so that, from the outside, it may seem as if you are looking at different minerals. But in the crystal kingdom, it's the internal structure or lattice that determines how we classify it.

The atoms and molecules that make up crystals are tightly packed; the pressure of the electromagnetic force of the earth leaves no space to be wasted in their makeup. The most efficient way to pack atoms into solid matter is an organized system of repeating shapes. The repeating shape is known as a unit cell. The internal structures of cubic crystal systems are made up of repeating unit cells stacked on top of and adjacent to each other.

Seven geometric shapes are used for crystal classification: square, rectangle, hexagon, triangle, rhombus, parallelogram, and trapezium. If you were to throw a crystal with force at the ground, you would see that it breaks into a similar shape with similar edges. So smoky quartz and calcite, both trigonal in makeup, would break in triangular shapes; sodalite, with its cubic arrangement, would shatter into square pieces. Crystals with a lattice break into smaller, similar shapes because of their strong, interlocking, repeating internal geometric structure.

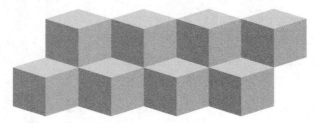

Example of a cubic crystal lattice

Amorphous minerals, however, are an exception to the rule. Where the geometric crystalline structures have order, amorphous minerals lack an organized internal structure. This occurs when a crystal's formation process is too fast, lacking time for the atoms to organize themselves in an ordered fashion as it rapidly coagulates into solid matter. It could also be that there are too many different substances that come together to form the rock.

Since shungite is classified as an amorphous metamorphic mineral, by definition it would lack any kind of organized internal structure. But one of the reasons why shungite is so special is that it's been found to be made up of fullerenes, also known as C_{60}, or carbon 60. Fullerenes are composed of twelve pentagonal and twenty hexagonal faces, which exist together in their molecular makeup to form a geodesic-dome-like structure reminiscent of a soccer ball.

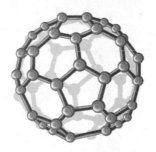

Named after the futurist and inventor Buckminster Fuller, who patented the geodesic domes made famous by the 1967 World's Fair in Montreal and Disney World's Epcot Center, this type of molecule wasn't discovered until 1985 by scientists Robert Curl, Harold Kroto, and Richard Smalley, who would go on to win the Nobel Prize in Chemistry in 1996 for their discovery.

Inspired by Kroto's theory that long carbon chains existed in the atmospheres of stars, this team of scientists conducted experiments designed to simulate the gas flow emanating from aging, carbon-rich stars. In doing so, they created an artificial, synthesized structure in their laboratory that seemed alien to earth's atmosphere. Because the extremely high temperatures and carefully controlled gas pressures needed to create fullerenes were so precise, it was believed that only a laboratory could house these perfect fullerene-making conditions. In 1992, though, natural fullerenes were accidentally discovered in shungite by geochemists at Arizona State University at Tempe[2] using a high-resolution transmission electron microscope, an instrument capable of recording images of individual molecules. In essence, humans had "created" a molecule that already existed; it just hadn't been discovered in nature yet.

Why is this important? Because understanding the structure of a crystal also helps us to understand why and how it works; in shungite, it's the fullerenes in particular that allow it to be so effective in absorbing EMFs as well as anxiety, which we'll look at in more depth in Chapters Four and Seven.

THE FORMATION OF SHUNGITE

Now that you are familiar with a few of these terms, you'll have a better understanding of what makes shungite so unique and important.

To understand the origins of shungite, we have to go back to our planet's formation story. It's believed that water-rich meteorites hit Earth's surface as the crust was carving itself out, which introduced the first water into Earth's atmosphere.

---

2 Malcolm W. Browne, "Nature, It Turns Out, Made a Molecule Long before People Did," *New York Times*, July 10, 1992.

Water condensation allowed the earliest elements of life to be introduced to the planet.

These first life forms, which evolved 3.8 billion years ago, were prokaryotes, cells that lack a nucleus or organized internal structure. They did, however, contain what's since been considered the origin of life: a single strand of DNA. Feeding on carbon compounds that accumulated in the early oceans, bacteria ultimately formed. These organisms developed to use the sun's energy and sulfides to generate their own energy, creating cyanobacteria, what we know today as blue-green algae, Earth's first oxygen producers by way of photosynthesis. Over time, enough oxygen accumulated in Earth's atmosphere to allow for the evolution of oxygen-metabolizing organisms, helping to jump-start the evolution of new, more complicated life.

Evolution didn't happen overnight, though. It took roughly 1–1.5 billion years for prokaryotes to develop into eukaryotes, cells with a defined nucleus and organelles. Talk about a glacial pace.

Shungite formed about 2.2 billion years ago. It consists of decomposed prokaryotes mixed with mud and silt to form kerogen, now the most abundant form of organic matter on Earth. These sediments slowly sank into the soil and, due to Earth's pressure, were compressed and transformed into rock. Geothermal heat and subterranean volcanic activity caused the organic materials to liquefy, transforming them further into simpler substances: hydrocarbons in the form of petroleum or bituminous shale and coal. This fluid spread out over 3,475 miles of land in what's considered today to be the Russian part of Karelia (the Karelia region straddles the border of Finland and northwest Russia), eventually forming shungite through the petrification process. Scientists believe that the petrification process allowed the natural molecular structure of fullerenes to form.

Because of their unique molecular structure, fullerenes, one of several classifications of carbon allotropes, are used as antiviral agents. An allotrope is an element, like the carbon in fullerenes, that can configure itself in such a way that its structure and properties change, even though its composition remains the same. Fullerenes' unique cage-like structures allow them to both carry needed molecules and trap dangerous substances in the body, and then to remove them. This makes shungite very effective in reducing the amount of electromagnetic radiation in and around a certain space.

In fact, research has shown that fullerenes are particularly potent in combating the flu,[3] inhibiting HIV-1 replication,[4] and suppressing herpes and other viral infections resistant to existing drugs.[5]

Why are these cage-like structures so efficient at trapping dangerous substances? Because of their high carbon makeup.

3   Masaki Shoji et al., "Anti-Influenza Activity of C_{60} Fullerene Derivatives," *PLoS One* 8, no. 6 (2013): e66337, https://www.ncbi.nlm.nih.gov/pmc/articles/ PMC3681905.
4   Zachary S. Martinez et al., "Fullerene Derivatives Strongly Inhibit HIV-1 Replication by Affecting Virus Maturation without Impairing Protease Activity," *Antimicrobial Agents and Chemotherapy* 60, no. 10 (2016): 5731–5741, https://aac.asm.org/ content/60/10/5731.
5   Regina Klimova et al., "Aqueous Fullerene C_{60} Solution Suppresses Herpes Simplex Virus and Cytomegalovirus Infections," *Fullerenes, Nanotubes and Carbon Nanostructures* 28, no. 6 (2020): 487–499, https://doi.org/10.1080/1536383X.2019.1706495.

Considered the magic of life, carbon is necessary for all life-forms. All living organisms contain carbon; it exists in nearly every compound in our bodies and every function our bodies carry out. We need it to live, grow, and reproduce. Carbon is especially unique in its ability to bond to other carbon molecules, as well as to form up to four covalent bonds between atoms or molecules. A covalent bond occurs when two atoms or molecules share an electron, enabling the atoms or molecules to stick together, which also stabilizes and strengthens them.

Electron-deficient in nature, fullerenes react easily with free radicals—unstable atoms that can damage cells, proteins, and DNA. Acting as antioxidants—molecules that neutralize free radicals—fullerenes' cage-like structure attracts and traps the free radicals and then transforms them into a neutral compound. This ability has made fullerenes popular in cosmetics technology as an anti-aging and anti-damage agent.

CHAPTER 2

The History and Healing Properties of Shungite

For as long as humans have walked this earth we've had a relationship with stones. To understand why we continue to be fascinated by them today—and why we're particularly enamored with shungite—we need to look back on our history with stones.

Planet Earth is about 4.5 billion years old; humans have only been walking it for about 2.5 million. But we didn't just hit the ground running with the knowledge we have today. It was learned over time. We had different skill sets, different burdens, different life-threatening fears that we as a species learned how to live with, grow from, and teach our offspring in a simpler, ancient world.

The relationship humans formed with stone has allowed us to evolve into the way of life we know today. In fact, human history is dated in periods based on the stone technology we relied on at the time: the Stone Age, the Bronze Age, and the Iron Age. At some point we realized that stones with sharp edges could be shaped into tools as well as weapons, to serve and protect. This revelation allowed us to overcome physical weakness and shape our environment, helping us to eventually give up the nomadic hunter-gatherer lifestyle with the technology needed to safeguard ourselves, settle down, and build communities.

Observing how their benefits directly affected our daily lives, we began to develop a reverence for these objects that helped us do so much. Soon we were incorporating stones into religions, regarding certain varieties as magic or sacred. We created altars out of stone to worship our gods, as a place to leave offerings and make sacrifices. These symbolic gestures point to an important shift in human development, signifying the first time our species did something that wasn't purely for survival. It was decorative and exemplified a belief in forces outside of ourselves that were thought to guide and assist our lives.

Stone was also seen as protective: its resistance to the elements solidified its importance in death rituals, the reason why tombstones, grave markers, and mausoleums continue to play an important part in our death rituals today.

Stones with holes in them were thought to be magical. Take the Men-an-Tol and Tolvan megaliths located in southwestern England, for example. It's now believed that babies and anyone who could fit through each stone's hole (20 inches and 17 inches wide, respectively) were passed through to help heal any sickness or ailment that had fallen upon them.

The first pieces of known jewelry were stones with holes in them, worn as bracelets or as necklaces. Jewelry then became not just a protective mechanism but an adornment and a status symbol.

The Sumerians settled in Mesopotamia, the "land between two rivers," the Tigris and Euphrates, as early as the fourth millennium BC. Their civilization is considered one of the earliest known to exist. Archaeological findings prove that the Sumerians believed certain precious stones and gems to be "miracle stones" that could ward off illness, attract love, and even protect the wearer from thieves.

The *Book of the Dead*, the infamous Egyptian text that details spells to navigate the afterlife, and uncovered tombs offer evidence that the Egyptians reached for different stones for different energies or purposes, such as protection, health, wisdom, and luck. It's believed that the Egyptians didn't name their crystals but classified them according to color, assigning each to different moods, which could be why we continue to associate anger with red and green with envy. This was most likely the inspiration behind mood rings, which first became popular in the 1970s. But the Egyptians also associated colors with different attributes of their gods. Thus, a stone's magical power was derived from the divine origin associated with it: red stones were from the blood of the gods; yellow stones an extension of the gods' skin; blue, their hair.

Persia was one of the first civilizations to adorn its kings with gems and jewelry in consecration ceremonies. Ancient Assyrian texts reveal that incantations were recited when creating "ornaments" for the kings to infuse the ruler with the energy of the gods and offer protection.

After winning the Persian War, the Greeks adopted the Persians' ideas that certain gems and crystals harnessed secret powers, which would go on to influence not only Greek architecture but also the culture and literature of the Hellenistic and late-classical eras.

In Rome, certain rules and rituals were put in place solely to utilize the magic inside a stone. At this time stones were "given souls" through specific formulas in order to unlock their magical potential; crystals "talked" to their owners. But should the owner let the crystal fall to the ground, its magic would be lost. If consecrated, the stone was meant to be worn at all times, but touching it or allowing it to make contact with the dead would pollute it.

Some of the ideas that the Romans lived by are still practiced today. One of the most popular ways to determine which crystal is for you is by the way it feels, or how it "speaks" to you. If you feel drawn to one specifically, it's considered a sign that that crystal is meant for you. And if your crystals come into contact with others, whether a friend picks one up or it's used in a group or healing session, some consider it to be "polluted," and it must be cleansed before it's practiced with again to dispel any energy that isn't yours.

Crystals continue to be utilized for their believed healing abilities today, whether placed directly on bodies, worn as jewelry, or doing double duty as both decor and space cleansers in homes. We'll talk more about how to use shungite in your everyday life for its healing abilities in the upcoming chapters, but for now let's focus on how shungite was discovered.

DISCOVERING SHUNGITE'S HEALING PROPERTIES

Surviving petroglyphs and rock paintings prove that many ancient peoples settled at Lake Onega, home of the largest deposit of shungite on Earth. They invite us into a culture directly connected to nature, the seasons, and the elements. Through archaeological digs, several sacred sites (labyrinths, sacred stones, and burial sites dating back to 6000 BC) have been unearthed in this area, which suggests that this was considered sacred territory. It's thought that the Sámi, an indigenous people of northern Europe whose traditional spiritual practice was based on animism—the notion that objects, places, and creatures all possess a distinct spiritual essence or soul—were among Lake Onega's early inhabitants because of the power they felt from the land.

In the fourteenth century, numerous Orthodox churches began to crop up in this area, their locations decided by trade routes and the sacred sites of the Sámi's ancestors so that the churches might be able to harness the same energetic properties.

The first mention of shungite's healing powers appears in writing from the seventeenth century. Boris Godunov, brother-in-law of Fyodor I and advisor to Ivan the Terrible, elected himself tsar in 1598 after the death of Fyodor, who left no heirs, ending the reign of the Rurik dynasty. In an attempt to keep his legitimacy to the throne from being challenged (because he was elected and not an actual heir), he banished the Romanovs, a noble family related to Fyodor I. Of them, Fyodor Nikitich Romanov, his wife Xenia, and their son Mikhail were exiled; Fyodor was sent to Poland; Xenia was sent to Tolvuya, north of Lake Onega, where she became a nun and assumed Martha as her name; and Mikhail was sent to Beloozero, then later was left in the care of other relatives. Because many knew who Martha was and why she was there, no one tried to help her when she became sick from the cold with little to keep her fed and warm.

It wasn't until 1605, when Boris Godunov died and his oppressive regime began to lift, that local peasants took pity on her, caring for her with water from the shungite spring. They boasted that it had miraculous properties. It did. Martha regained her health and was able to reunite with her son, who, in 1613, elected himself tsar, returning the Romanov family back to the throne and thus founding the Romanov dynasty. The spring from which Martha was thought to have regained her health was renamed the Spring of the Princess.

The healing powers of shungite wouldn't gain attention again until the reign of Peter the Great, much later in the eighteenth century. Legend has it that workers in a copper factory located near Lake Onega fell ill, showing signs of poison, but they regained their health and strength after drinking "living water" from a nearby spring. When news of this mysterious healing made its way to St. Petersburg, Peter the Great ordered an investigation of this obscure spring, which poured out from a shungite deposit. People saw a direct correlation when those who had scurvy, liver problems, and other ailments drank water from this particular spring and miraculously seemed to recover.

Peter the Great had been on a healing quest of his own. His doctor had sent him to the original thermal spa in Belgium (we get the word *spa* from the name of the Belgian town Spa) for one month to help cure his liver ailments. This tsar was particularly keen on having a spa with its own proven healing powers to rival that of Belgium. To put Russia on the map as a healing destination, he ordered the construction of the first Russian spa to exploit the medicinal properties of shungite. Thus, Russia's first-ever spa, Marcial Waters, was built on the shores of a small lake near Lake Onega.

The famous tsar frequented the spa with his family and, having experienced a sense of renewed vitality from shungite's purifying effect on the water, commanded that every Russian soldier carry a piece of shungite (then referred to as "slate rock") at all times. He believed this would give them constant access to pure, disinfected water, helping them to avoid dysentery, a highly contagious intestinal infection that plagued armies at that particular time in history.

Though it was first used as a magical elixir for a leaky gut, more recent studies and research on shungite prove that it has many other healing properties. For instance, it:

• Aids in cellular regeneration

• Is considered yin, receptive energy

- Demonstrates anti-inflammatory properties

- Fights and neutralizes toxins in the body

- Harmonizes and rebalances energy

- Helps stabilize blood pressure

- Improves sleep

- Increases enzymatic activity

- Neutralizes electromagnetic fields, significantly weakening the effects of EMFs on the human body

- Possesses antibacterial qualities

- Promotes the exchange of information between neurotransmitters

- Protects from both ionizing and non-ionizing radiation

- Purifies and energizes water

- Restores emotional balance to help alleviate anxiety, depression, and stress

- Speeds up healing of wounds

- Stimulates tissue regeneration

- Strengthens immunity

- Treats digestive illnesses

- Works as one of the most powerful free radical–fighting antioxidants

Shungite's antioxidant properties and unique fullerene makeup have proven to be helpful in reducing psoriasis, acne, signs of aging, and other skin conditions when used topically. Because of this, it's now being used in Russian skin-care lines and beauty products.

Shungite's anti-inflammatory properties allow it to help relieve pain in the form of headaches, migraines, back and joint pain, rheumatism, and osteoarthritis. It's also helpful for digestive illnesses like gastritis, colitis, pancreatitis, and acid reflux, and it reduces bloating and aids in elimination issues like chronic constipation or diarrhea.

Because of its natural ability to reduce the effects of EMFs, which can unbalance our own energy and increase anxiety, shungite has also been shown to soothe insomnia and other sleep issues.

Now that you have a better understanding of what shungite is capable of, we'll take a look at how its shape affects how its energy is focused, some simple ways to incorporate the mineral in your home to maximize its potential, and more complex practices to improve your health using shungite as an energetic antidote.

CHAPTER 3

Amplify Your Energy Using Shungite

Science has been slow to explain energetic phenomena, to disclose the reasons why we react and respond to certain stimuli and not others, but finally we have answers to some of our most burning questions. What a gift it is to have studies backing the claims of what many of us have believed in without question for thousands of years. Our ancestors didn't offer scientific arguments to back their use of certain crystals for specific healing outcomes. Instead they connected to the minerals they incorporated into their healing rituals and trusted what they felt in order to understand the specific energetic properties of each. They understood that there are many things invisible to the naked eye that affect us energetically as well as on a cellular level. The healings our ancestors oversaw were successful because they believed them to be effective and so they were, not just because the effects of their treatments were compelling, but because they believed in the crystals' powers.

In this chapter we'll look at ways and practices in which you can use shungite to support your physical, mental, and emotional well-being. Some of you may experience noticeable differences in how you feel, others may only notice subtle shifts, and still others may not experience anything at all.

Belief and expectation play significant roles when working with crystals. If this book is in your hands, you likely already believe or want to believe they can enhance or help our lives. If you believe or are open to the idea that incorporating any of these practices can assist you, then they will make a difference. If you are closed off to the possibility that communing with crystals can assist your health, then these practices might not do as much for you.

Note: *When you acquire your first pieces of shungite, you will want to sit with or near them for small periods of time as you start to acclimate to their energy and power. Being too close to them for too long when you first start to work with shungite can bring on headaches and nausea for the energetically sensitive.*

SHAPES

Raw pieces are natural specimens that come from the earth and tend to have a ragged, unpolished appearance and a strong and sporadic energy.

Recommended use: Small raw pieces or chips are great to use in drinking water, in a bath, or in an aura spray. You'll find instructions on how to make these items in the following pages.

Tumbled stones are typically small raw pieces that have been polished to have smooth surfaces and have a gentle, even energy.

Recommended use: Worn as jewelry or kept on your person in a pocket, tucked away in your bra or anywhere else your clothing allows you to hold a small object close to your body/skin. Wearing a shungite pendant on a necklace to cover your heart or throat chakras offers a way to accessorize while protecting these energy centers. You can also wear shungite bracelets, earrings, and rings. All have grounding, protective effects.

Spheres are pieces that have been polished into a perfectly round shape and give off a smooth, pulsing energy evenly in all directions. Spheres have long been associated with crystal balls and scrying, tools to help you see into the future. Shungite spheres specifically help clear blockages around the sixth and seventh chakras, the third eye, and our connection to higher wisdom.

Recommended use: Hold one in either hand while meditating, or keep on your altar or desk.

Harmonizers are cylindrical pieces that have been polished to have a smooth surface with flat ends. Often sold in pairs, one looks black in color while the other seems more like a dusty gray. The black harmonizer is shungite and the other is usually steatite, a metamorphic rock that promotes positivity as it helps soothe and balance your energy.

Recommended use: Hold the black shungite harmonizer in the left hand and the steatite in the right hand while meditating. Shungite is more yin, receptive energy, which is associated with our left side. Steatite is more yang, active energy, commonly associated with the right side.

Towers or **generators** have six facets that meet at a point, which helps focus and amplify the properties of the crystal.

Recommended use: Ideal for crystal grids, a pattern or setup of crystals that helps amplify and direct energy toward your intention.

Pyramids give off a highly focused energy to clear negative or unwanted energy and remove blockages. The larger the pyramid, the larger its range of effectiveness.

Recommended use: Place in areas where you spend lots of time: under your bed, under your couch, or on your desk near your computer. They can also be used as a centerpiece in grids.

Cubes have a very grounding and stabilizing energy.

Recommended use: Place in all four corners of a room full of electronics to add a protective, stabilizing energy.

SHUNGITE AT WORK

Buyer Beware: While shungite can be a godsend to help protect yourself from EMFs, sometimes it performs too well. There have been numerous reports of people trying to use it to neutralize the electromagnetic fields in or around their homes, only to have issues with their electronics working properly.

Over time, you may also notice a white line appear on your shungite. This doesn't happen with every piece, but rest assured that should yours suddenly take on a stripe it's just a sign that it's hard at work. Think of it like Rogue's infamous battle with Magneto in the first X-Men movie: Rogue's character has the ability to absorb and sometimes even remove memories, superpowers, physical strength, and even personality traits when she makes skin-to-skin contact with another person. Magneto tries to harvest her superpower at the end of the movie and, in self-preservation, Rogue's powers try to fight the radiation given off by Magneto's machine—meant to give humans superpowers and strip mutants of their own. As she uses everything she has to protect herself, a white streak appears in her hair because of the force she's had to exert to fight off the radiation. It's for this same reason that your shungite might suddenly display some highlights (minus the fight scene). It just means it's doing what it's meant to.

 ## CRYSTAL ELIXIR

One of the first ways shungite's healing properties were ever utilized was via drinking water. Since shungite's antioxidant properties help it absorb metals and neutralize contaminants found in water, making your own crystal elixir with shungite is an effective way to filter and purify your drinking water while also infusing it with oxygen, calcium, and magnesium. Plus, it's a direct way to absorb shungite's energy to help the body fight off harmful free radicals, increasing your metabolism and improving skin quality. Shungite's ability to reactivate and revitalize enables the water to hydrate the body on a deeper, more powerful level.

Note: *To create this special elixir, you will want to use elite shungite.*

1. For every 34-ounce pitcher of shungite water you make, you will need about 2–3 ounces of elite shungite. Depending on the size of your shungite, you could use anywhere from two to five pieces.

2. Clean your shungite. Use your hands or a brush to gently scrub away black residue, mud, and any other impurities with filtered water. Do not use soap.

3. Place the shungite in a glass pitcher and fill with water.

4. Let sit for anywhere from 6 to 24 hours, avoiding direct sunlight. The longer your shungite water sits, the better the results.

5. Once consumed, keep the shungite you used in the pitcher and refill with water to create your next batch.

Note: *The first time you drink shungite water, start small: only consume about a highball's worth of liquid. Just as you need to get used to its feel and develop a tolerance to the pieces you buy for your home, your body also needs time to adjust and build a tolerance to this powerful new substance. You can increase the size of your beverage over time.*

This crystal elixir is also safe and beneficial for your pets to drink and for watering plants; you can also use it to cook with, brew coffee, or make tea.

You may also consider introducing shungite water into your self-care and beauty regimens to wash your face or hands; the free radical–fighting fullerenes found in shungite have been connected with speeding up the process of cell regeneration, helping to calm acne and other skin issues and working as an anti-aging agent.

> **Pro tip:** *Cleanse the pieces you use in your pitcher by taking them out of your pitcher and setting them in the sun every four to six months. Clean your pitcher once a month, or whenever a milky residue starts to appear on the glass.*

MINERAL BATH

You can also access the benefits of shungite water by enjoying a shungite bath. Immersing yourself in shungite water is great for hypertension, joint pain, circulation illnesses, and psoriasis and other skin issues. It also helps reduce fatigue, reinvigorating your whole body.

Place a few pieces of elite shungite in a full bath and let sit for about 10 minutes before getting in. Then luxuriate in the bath for up to 20 minutes before getting out.

GRIDS

At its most basic, a grid really only needs two things: crystals and an intention.

Let's first talk crystals: There is no limit to the number of crystals you use to create your grid, but you must use a minimum of two crystals for it to be considered a grid. One specific crystal can speak to you and be powerful by itself, but when combining other pieces in a grid, the interaction they have and the power they create between them transcends what just one crystal can do or is capable of.

Think about any job you've ever had at an established business. Your role, whether you were a waiter, an actor, a writer, a teacher, or a truck driver, was important on its own; without you, certain things just would not have been done. But your job along with everyone else's enhanced the overall performance and potential of your place of business. Everyone's roles complemented each other to make the whole business strong and functional. Similarly, the energy of a grid is greater than the energy of the individual crystals: working together, they magnify each other's energy.

Next, you need an intention. A grid makes for great decor or a conversational piece in your home, but without a clear and specific intention, the energy created by the grid has nowhere to direct itself. Crystal grids can help us to build up and strengthen our energy while helping us to rewire the parts of our personal energy fields that were weak or we lacked access to, but we need to tell the grid where we are directing the energy.

Disney's Cinderella sang: "A dream is a wish your heart makes, when you're fast asleep." An intention, on the other hand, is a conscious wish your heart and mind make, an opportunity to call in support from the universe to invite in something specific to assist you on your path.

Intentions can be set for anything, but since we're talking about shungite specifically, here are some themes that can be especially dynamic when creating a shungite grid:

- Abundance

- Alleviating anxiety, depression, or stress

- Aura strengthening

- Breaking through obstacles

- Chakra balancing

- Energetic protection

- Enhancing intuition

- Health and vitality

- Improved sleep

- Personal growth

- Purification of body, mind, and spirit

- Transcending physical pain

When you set an intention, it is best phrased as extremely specific and in the first person, as if you already are living it. Here are a few shungite-specific examples:

- I fall asleep easily and sleep soundly through the night

- I feel strong and healthy in my body

- My energy is strong; it communicates and flows freely within me

- My strong connection to my intuition helps me make decisions that are in the highest and best interest for me and all those around me

Think of your intention like a love letter to yourself. Many people think that intention-setting or manifestation work is about bringing in something physical that you don't already have: objects, money, a person, love, a new career, a new home. And while manifestation work can certainly bring about these things eventually, it's really about calling in the *feeling* of what you're hoping to call in, the feeling you are unable to connect with regularly. First, connect to the why of what you are trying to call in: Why do I want this? How will this benefit my life? Why is this important to me?

After you've got your why, next you have to connect with the feeling of having what you're trying to manifest. Don't try to paint what life will look like after you've achieved your intention; instead focus on what it feels like to fully embody it. The crystals in your grid will help anchor you into this feeling.

In terms of setting up your grid, think of it like an arts and crafts project: figure out which crystals you would like to use and what energies you want to amplify your intention. Even if you don't remember the names of the other crystals you own or their properties, the power of your grid lies in the trust you have for yourself as you figure out what looks and feels good together.

Some people like to use numerology to help them set up their grids, while others look to sacred geometry. And while both of these tools can be helpful, having a knowledge of either is not necessary to create a potent grid. You have an innate connection to yourself and the energy of the crystals you are using; even if you aren't sure of the meaning behind using three crystals versus seven, if you set up your grid in a way that *feels* right to you, you will never be wrong. Let your intuition be your guide, and allow yourself to have fun while setting them up.

Your grids don't have to be big or complicated. They can be simple. A grid can have a hundred crystals in it, or it can just have two. Whenever there are two or more crystals together, they are in communication with each other energetically. So start with two and play around with their placement, including how far apart you'd like to set them from each other. Shift their orientation so you get a feel for them in relation to the different sides (front, back, left, right, top, bottom) they can show to one another. As you add or take away stones, the feel of the grid will change, too. Add more to your design if you feel called to do so; keep it as is if you don't.

You can create grids using just one type of crystal, or you can incorporate all different types. It's completely up to you. You can elect to place a crystal at the center of your grid as a focal point, or not. But know this: the center stone of a crystal grid works like the heart in the toroidal field (which we'll discuss more in Chapter Six), where energy is both received (in the form of your intention) and broadcasted out; the energy sent out by your crystal grid is healing. Having a centerpiece shifts the energy of the entire grid, so play around with your setup and trust what feels right.

Everyone is different and has different needs, feels energy differently, and has different relationships with their crystals and minerals. As you embark on your shungite journey you can use the protection grid described below and the suggestions listed in Chapter Six as a jumping-off place to build from as you create grids in your home, or you can flex your intuitive muscle to create something unique that feels right to you.

However you choose to proceed, know this: there is no wrong way to build a grid. The possibilities are limitless.

Note: *Size matters. The larger a piece, the further its range can travel. If shungite isn't already part of your crystal collection, opt for one that's a decent size to place in your home or to use for gridwork. If you have a small piece of shungite but have a large clear quartz crystal, you can place the shungite on top of the quartz to magnify the shungite's energy.*

 PROTECTION GRID

Harnessing the protective qualities of shungite, this grid is an effective way to shield yourself from the negative energy of coworkers, family members, or anyone you may encounter who makes you feel uneasy.

1. Place a pyramid or tower of shungite in the center.

2. Surround the centerpiece with three pointed shungite pieces. Use pyramids or towers or a mix of the two.

3. Connect the outside pieces to the centerpiece by placing smaller crystals in between.

4. If you have large clear or smoky quartz pieces, feel free to add them to enhance the energy of the grid, placing them wherever they feel right and balanced to you.

5. Write your intention on a piece of paper, fold it up, and place it under the centerpiece.

Sample intentions to use with your protection grid:

- My boundaries are strong with [insert name of person you want protection from]

- I have the strength and courage necessary to stand up for myself

- I am protected from negative energy

 SHUNGITE JOURNAL

A great way to track any changes or shifts in your life once you start working with this powerful mineral is to keep a shungite journal. It's recommended to keep a tumbled piece of shungite with you at all times. Larger pieces are also welcome for the first step. Here is an idea to help get you started:

1. Take a few moments to close your eyes and notice how you feel physically, mentally, and emotionally before picking up your specimen. Write down how you feel.

2. Next, hold your shungite in your hands and close your eyes. Again, notice how you feel physically, mentally, and emotionally while holding your crystal. Write down these new feelings.

Do this check-in every day to help you see the immediate ways shungite affects your energy. Use your journal to record when you do something new or seemingly out of character as a means of protection (e.g., feeling emboldened to stand up for yourself, deciding to disengage from a negative conversation, removing yourself from an uncomfortable situation, etc.). Celebrate yourself for the hard work and courage it took for you to shift your behavior.

Remember that evolution happens slowly, but taking the time to write down your thoughts and insights on your progress will help you see how just the simple act of carrying shungite with you can help you strengthen so many different areas of your life at once. Seeing your growth in writing will help you feel more empowered to try new things and take risks, helping you to break through your energetic blocks and transform your life.

◇◇◇

Shifting your energy can be hard, but utilizing the powerhouse mineral shungite to assist you on your healing journey can help support and enhance your health, vitality, and overall life experience and find ease in all your transitions. What follows is an in-depth look at how modern-day dilemmas affect us physically, emotionally, and energetically; why and how employing shungite in our homes and healing rituals can help us manage our physical and mental health; and several suggested practices to use shungite to help enhance your personal energy.

CHAPTER 4

Everything You Need to Know about EMFs

Before we start talking about EMFs, let's review some basic science about our friend the atom, just so we're all on the same page.

An atom is the basic unit of a chemical element, made up of protons (the positive charge), neutrons (neutral charge), and electrons (negative charge). The protons and neutrons live together in the center of the atom, called the nucleus, and lend the atom most of its mass; electrons fly around the nucleus, orbiting in a small cloud. The number of protons an atom contains determines the type of atom it is. If you look at the periodic table, the number at the top of each box refers to the number of protons each element contains.

A molecule is a group of two or more atoms.

While it was once thought that electrons orbited the nucleus much like the moon orbits the Earth, it's been found that electrons are best described as wave functions, acting more like force fields that surround and protect the protons and neutrons. The number of electrons an atom contains is equal to the number of protons in its nucleus.

Chemical reactions can sometimes strip away an electron or even invite more in. When this happens, the modified atom is called an ion. When an atom has more electrons than protons, the atom gains a negative charge; these are negative ions. When there are more protons than electrons, a positive ion is created.

The human electromagnetic field (the aura, which we'll talk more about in the next chapter) is made up of both positive and negative ions. Negative ions are found in abundance in nature: the mountains, the ocean, waterfalls, or after a good rain. It's because of this affluence of negative ions that it feels so refreshing, energizing, and invigorating to be in these areas and conditions. When inhaled or absorbed into the bloodstream, it's believed that negative ions produce biochemical reactions that increase levels of the mood enhancer serotonin, which helps alleviate depression, relieve stress, and boost your energy.

Positive ions, on the other hand, can be energetically depleting, draining you of your energy, making you feel tired and lethargic, and contributing to feelings of tension, anxiety, and irritability. Positive ions occur naturally, formed by strong winds, dust, humidity, and pollution. They also are a byproduct of electrical appliances.

ELECTRIC CURRENTS

There are two types of electric current: AC, or alternating current, and DC, direct current. And yes, this is exactly where the band AC/DC gets its name.

AC charges move in two different directions, alternating between them in pulses. DC only flows in one direction. Because the earth creates a DC magnetic charge and electric field, DC currents are what we experience in nature. It's also the current that the body uses to send signals throughout itself, making it possible for us to move, think, and feel.

Electricity is the flow of electrons between atoms; voltage is what pushes the electrons around a circuit. Voltage is defined as the potential difference (how much work can possibly be done through a circuit) in charge between two points in an electrical field. Without voltage, the free electrons will still move around atoms, but randomly. It's only when voltage is applied that the electrons will move in the same direction, causing current, the flow of electrons in a circuit.

An electromagnetic field (EMF) is the invisible area of energy produced by electricity, created by stationary or moving electric charge. A stationary charge produces an electric field in the surrounding space, but if the charge is moving, a magnetic field is also created. To help explain the difference between the two, let's think about your TV.

When your TV is off, it's still plugged into the wall, still connected to an electric source, still possessing the ability to move energy through its wiring. The outlet, the cord running from the TV to the outlet, and the television are giving off an electric field even though the power isn't turned on.

When the TV is on, electricity is passed through the cord and the wires within the cord to allow the TV to function. When an electric current is moving, when energy is in motion, a magnetic field exists.

Electric fields can be present if there is no magnetic field, but magnetic fields can only exist if an electric field is present.

All living beings are considered to be electromagnetic: electrical currents run through the human body and are considered essential for life. The nervous system requires electricity to send signals to the brain and throughout the body that make it possible to move, think, and feel. Even our emotions have frequencies: they carry voltage, pushing energy through us. Elements of the human body are also piezoelectric. Piezoelectricity is the electrical current produced when mechanical stress or mechanical excitation is applied to the human body, or any object (including crystals and audio speakers).

DNA and bone have long been known to produce currents within themselves when a mechanical stress or excitation is applied to the body. A study titled "Piezoelectricity in the Human Pineal Gland," conducted in 1996, found not only that tissues in the pineal gland are piezoelectric, but also that, more importantly, the pineal gland itself could respond to EMFs, proving that the human body, indeed, is affected by

EMFs.[6] (The pineal gland sits directly behind the amygdala in the brain; it's responsible for secreting melatonin—the hormone that helps you sleep—into the bloodstream. We'll talk about the pineal gland at length in Chapter Five when we discuss the chakras.)

WHY YOU SHOULD CARE ABOUT EMFS

As technology has evolved over time and you rely more and more on devices that require electricity and fill your home, you are constantly surrounded by various forms of EMFs. Take a look around at the things you have to plug in, in order for them to work: lamps, refrigerators, computers, toasters, ovens, chargers, radios, gaming consoles, hair dryers, electric toothbrushes, diffusers, fitness trackers, printers, white noise machines, fans, and other random devices not listed here that are unique to your tastes and needs.

To an extent, you can control the number of electromagnetic fields in your home by turning things off or unplugging devices when you're not using them. But in this day and age, Wi-Fi has become ubiquitous, one of the most important necessities of modern life. It provides streaming services for all your internet needs: it likely offers you at least one or two television services (Netflix, Hulu, Amazon Prime Video, Fios, Roku, etc.); allows your smartphone to be, well, smart; powers game consoles like PlayStation, Xbox, and Nintendo;

---

6   Sidney B. Lang et al., "Piezoelectricity in the Human Pineal Gland," *Bioelectrochemistry and Bioenergetics* 41, no. 2 (1996): 191–195, https://www.sciencedirect .com/science/article/abs/pii/ S0302459896051471.

and lets you download books to your Kindle. It's an invention of convenience. But unless you're turning your Wi-Fi router off at night when you go to bed and unplugging all the cords that power your electronics, you live in the presence of continuous magnetic fields.

It's important to note that a magnetic field is strongest at the source; its power decreases as you increase your distance from the source. Since magnetic fields can pass through buildings, living things, and most other materials, if you live in a city—especially apartment buildings or condominiums, places where there are many units located very close together—you're likely exposed to more magnetic fields than if you lived in an area where homes are more spread out.

Even if we gave up all our creature comforts, we wouldn't be able to completely hide from EMFs. No matter where you reside, there are bound to be power lines nearby. Think about where you live and how many utility poles accessorize your neighborhood and your street. No matter if you live in the city, the suburbs, or the country, you live in close proximity to magnetic fields, if not right smack-dab in the middle of them.

DIFFERENT TYPES OF EMFS

EMFs exist in two different forms: low-level radiation and high-level radiation. Low-level radiation is non-ionizing, which refers to any type of electromagnetic radiation that doesn't carry enough energy to ionize atoms or molecules—that is, to completely remove an electron from an atom or molecule. Electronic appliances like microwaves, cell phones, computers, TVs, Wi-Fi routers, Bluetooth devices, power lines, and MRIs are classified as low-level radiators.

High-level radiation, or ionizing radiation, is emitted by ultraviolet (UV) light rays from the sun and medical imaging devices like X-rays that easily pass through all tissues in the body. Remember when we mentioned ions earlier? Ionizing radiation has the unique capability to remove electrons from atoms and molecules in the matter through which it passes. This means it can actually alter molecules within the cells of our body, breaking the covalent bonds in our DNA and converting water found in the nucleus, where most DNA is stored, to hydroxyl free radicals, one of the most dangerous free radicals in the body. Hydroxyl radicals are unable to travel far, but since they are created in the nucleus, right next to your DNA, they are capable of breaks in both single and double strands. Because of its ability to affect humans on a cellular level, high-level radiation has been linked to causing skin, tissue, and genetic damage, as well as cancer.

Depending on the source, the amount of radiation a device gives off varies, but one rule is true: the closer you are to the source of an EMF-emitting mechanism, the more exposure you receive. Just as ultraviolet rays from the sun will be the strongest and most intense the closer you are to the equator, you'll be picking up more EMFs from your Apple Watch or smartphone if it is always on you or beside you than if it is in the next room.

The electromagnetic spectrum encompasses the entire range of EMF radiation, ranked from lowest to highest frequencies. Since EMF radiation travels in waves, the frequency refers to how many waves per second a source gives off.

The spectrum starts with longer, lower frequencies mostly from electrical sources that have been established to be non-ionizing, like power lines, radios and TVs, and cell phones. One radio wave can be as long as a football field. As you continue to progress across the spectrum, the waves become shorter as they move faster and their frequencies increase. Think microwaves, infrared devices, and visible light. (Microwave wavelengths measure approximately 12 centimeters.) The waves feel almost erratic in nature as their frequencies becomes stronger and faster, as with waves of ultraviolet radiation, X-rays, and radioactive waste. X-ray wavelengths measure between 0.01 and 10 nanometers; 1 nanometer is equal to one billionth of a meter.

Most of the devices we use on a regular basis sit in the safe zone of the electromagnetic spectrum, where frequencies are longer. They are classified "safe" because non-ionizing radiation from our cell phones, Wi-Fi, and other wireless accessories lack the energy to knock off electrons and damage DNA that ionizing radiation—such as UV rays, X-rays, and radioactive waste—is capable of. But research shows that non-ionizing radiation causes damage to our cells in a completely different way. Where ionizing radiation creates hydroxyl free radicals, non-ionizing radiation creates carbonyl free radicals that cause near-identical damage.

One of the major reasons there's controversy around the idea that non-ionizing radiation is harmful is that we've been told it's safe. We trust manufacturers to make smart, safe decisions on our behalf about the technology we use, but sometimes our vision of how these inventions can help make our lives easier, or our greed—or both!—push companies to get new devices on the market without fully understanding their effects on our health. For example: cigarettes, Styrofoam, and some plastics (such as polyethylene terephthalate, high-density polyethylene, polyvinyl chloride, low-density polyethylene, polypropylene, and bisphenol A) are very harmful. If we had known their effects on the planet and on our health, if we could have seen into the future to understand what life would look like after introducing these products into our lives and ecosystem, would we have ever produced them in the first place?

PERPETUALLY IN AWE OF ELECTRICITY

Since electricity's invention, we humans have been enamored by it, fixated on its magic. Even when it was first discovered, we were warned against its powers. But from the moment of its inception, we only saw what we wanted to see: that it was capable of untold wonders, that it could help us do the unimaginable. Most, so captivated with electricity's possibilities and how it could help make our lives easier, overlooked the warnings that were touted by those concerned with its effects on our health. We still have this relationship to it today.

EFFECTS OF EMFS ON THE BODY

Current safety tests of wireless devices put in place by the Federal Communications Commission (FCC), an independent agency of the US government that regulates communications by radio, television, wire, satellite, and cable across the US, only assess the amount of heat a device gives off. Heat is a byproduct of non-ionizing radiation: when radiation is present, it excites electrons into higher-energy orbitals around the nucleus. Eventually the electron returns to its nonexcited state; it's here that excess energy is released as heat from neighboring molecules, increasing the temperature of the system.

At present, there are no tests conducted by manufacturers on the effects that our internet-connected electronics have on human beings on a cellular level, where the damage is actually happening. Also, manufacturers' current testing protocols don't take into account where we might be using our devices; in places where our phones require more power and have to work harder to find a signal (rural areas, elevators, cars), we're more exposed. Note that said tests are also done on dummies and not actual living human beings. So testing lacks accuracy in a variety of ways.

The thing we have to understand about radiation is that just because we can't see it doesn't mean it's not there. Anything that is bad for us doesn't seem like it is the first few times we do it: sleeping too much or too little, eating fast food, not brushing your teeth, sitting all day, not getting enough exercise. But if we keep up these "bad" habits, over time we'll notice their effects on our health. In some cases we're able to shift our habits to regain our health; in others the damage is done and there is no turning back. The effects of EMF radiation aren't noticeable the first time you pick up a cell phone or the day you start working on a computer with wireless internet connectivity. EMF damage is only noticeable as it accumulates over time from regular exposure. We'll look at these symptoms and effects later in this chapter.

History has proven that we have a hard time understanding, respecting, or even believing in invisible forces around us that affect our health—even when the science is there.

Let's recall the 1986 Chernobyl disaster, an explosion of one of the reactors in the Ukrainian nuclear power plant. Though the effects of radiation happened much faster and were more excruciating if someone touched a piece of the graphite that had exploded from the reactor's core—as some of the firefighters who were first called in to help control the fires that raged in and around the sector experienced—an invisible threat hung in the air and ended up taking the lives of all the firefighters who showed up blind to and ignorant of the real enemy they were fighting, whether they made physical contact with the graphite or not.

The invisible threat was the nuclear radiation; within minutes of arriving on the scene, nearly every firefighter began to experience some form of radiation sickness. In the first few months following the accident thirty-one people died (twenty-seven of whom were firefighters); thousands more would eventually follow as cancers and tumors developed in locals from radiation exposure. The National Research Center for Radiation Medicine (NRCRM) estimates that close to six million citizens of the former USSR, including the Ukraine and Belarus, have suffered as a result of the radiation following the disaster.[7] About two million people continue to hold status as victims of the disaster today, and the number of disabilities within this population continue to rise.

There's no question that the invisible strength of the radiation emitted from the nuclear power plant affected not just millions, but generations, yet had it not caused such clear, physical damage to first responders and those in the immediate area (read: 1,000 square-mile exclusion zone), would we all have agreed on nuclear radiation's effects on the human body? Wildlife has begun to return to Chernobyl, and in 2011 authorities allowed the site to reopen to the public; tours of the abandoned nuclear site are all the rage today. But radiation levels are still ten to one hundred times higher than normal background radiation, and scientists estimate the zone around the former plant won't be habitable, according to Chernobyl power plant director Ihor Gramotkin, for up to twenty thousand years.

At the time of the explosion, when the horrors of nuclear radiation were still very much present, it was predicted it would be thousands of years until it was considered safe to return to the site. Now that tours are being led through the area to show a glimpse of the old USSR and the infamous abandoned nuclear power plant, tour company websites give explicit recommendations that visitors show up with

7   V. O. Sushko et al., "Problems of Medical Expertise for Diseases that Bring to Disability and Death as a Result of Radiation Exposure Influence in Conditions of the Chernobyl Catastrophe in Remote Postaccidental Period," *Problems of Radiation Medicine and Radiobiology* 23 (2018): 471–480, https://pubmed.ncbi.nlm.nih.gov/30582864.

dosimeters to measure the amount of radiation they are being exposed to. (Don't worry, they have some you can rent if you don't have your own.)

Similar to dosimeters, EMF meters are used by wireless service technicians when working on cell towers today. There is only so much EMF radiation—or any kind of radiation—the body can absorb before it begins to deteriorate. People who work in the industry use these devices to let them know when they've withstood the maximum radiation a body should be exposed to.

If we can believe that invisible nuclear radiation is harmful to the body, why is it a stretch to believe that invisible electromagnetic frequencies also are harmful to the body? Because again, we have a hard time believing in the "magic" of things we can't see, which also keeps many people from believing in the aura, the chakras, and even the power of crystals.

But the relationship between how much we use and rely on electricity and the resulting rise of chronic diseases cannot be overlooked.

Studies show that the closer you live to a cell phone tower, the more effects you notice on and in your body over time— in other words, the greater the amount of damage.[8] Since the strength of a magnetic field is most powerful at its source, think of cell phone towers as the queen bees: Because they

---

8   Thomas Haumann et al. "HF-Radiation Levels of GSM Cellular Phone Towers in Residential Areas," in *Biological Effects of EMFs: 2nd International Workshop (Rhodes, Greece, 7–11 October 2002); Proceedings*, ed. P. Kostarakis, vol. 1 (Ioannina, Greece: University of Ioannina, 2002), 327–333.

receive and transmit radio waves to all cell phones on the same network in the area, their magnetic fields are amplified to accommodate their range and reach. Even if you turned off your Wi-Fi routers at night, if you lived near a cell tower, your caution would be for naught: you'd still be in the vicinity of the most powerful EMFs.

DID YOU KNOW?

It's recommended that you hold your cell phone 5 to 15 millimeters away from your body while it's turned on to reduce your exposure to EMFs. The distance or range varies from model to model, but these recommendations come directly from your phone's manufacturer and are actually printed in your owner's manual, so you may want to dig yours up.

The average amount of time a person uses or looks at their phones is at an all-time high, with 96 percent of Americans owning at least one cell or smartphone, and sales continue to rise.[9] To handle this demand, existing cell phone towers need to be strengthened and new frequencies added; the total number of cell phone towers will only increase in order to meet our needs.

There are many websites you can visit in order to see where you live in relation to cell towers in your area. And while many people who experience electrohypersensitivity— noticeable side effects or symptoms from EMF radiation that

---

9   Pew Research Center, "Demographics of Mobile Device Ownership and Adoption in the United States," June 5, 2020, https://www.pewresearch.org/internet/factsheet/mobile.

include unexplained allergies, tinnitus (even in people with no prior ear injuries or problems), slowed mind function, memory loss, headaches, insomnia, depression, attention deficit hyperactivity disorder (ADHD), dizziness, nausea, intense tingling or burning sensations of the skin, irritability, restlessness, and anxiety—are already literally running for the hills (i.e., rural areas with less coverage), pretty soon, with the rollout of 5G technology, there will be no more hills to run to as the entire globe will be wirelessly linked; areas that once had no coverage will eventually be connected. So your boss can contact you anywhere in the world. And you'll be constantly exposed to electromagnetic radiation. Yay.

In *Better Call Saul*, the prequel spin-off of *Breaking Bad* that takes a look at how criminal lawyer Jimmy McGill becomes the crooked lawyer Saul Goodman in the hit TV series, Jimmy's older brother Chuck, played by *SNL* alum Michael McKean, is electrohypersensitive. He's disconnected his house from electricity, lines his walls with aluminum foil, shrouds himself in a space blanket, and makes Jimmy leave his cell phone in the mailbox whenever his brother comes to visit. His condition is so severe that he rarely leaves the house since electricity is everywhere. The show and its characters make Chuck out to seem like he's crazy, as if it's all in his head, and in doing so shed light on how many who suffer from electrohypersensitivity are treated or regarded.

Electrohypersensitivity is becoming more widely known, but many are still unaware of it. It's much more common than you think, but due to the stigma around it, often those affected don't talk about it openly—similar to how people didn't openly talk about anxiety until the last few decades. Those who notice a sensitivity to electricity report working or living near high-power electric lines or cell phone towers. As a result, they suffer from migraines, notice extreme joint inflammation, or feel sick or nauseated on a regular basis. Others notice dull aches or tingling sensations when their smartphone makes contact with their body, insomnia, neck pain, confusion, increased irritability when around electronics for prolonged periods of time, feeling scrambled or jittery after sitting in front of a computer for too long, and even hearing the buzz of electricity when devices are on.

Not that these symptoms do not or cannot exist on their own for other reasons, but many sufferers have learned about the benefits of using shungite and other EMF-fighting mechanisms to alleviate symptoms. These include Q-Link bracelets, Faraday cages (metallic enclosures that help shield whoever sits inside them from EMFs, while also preventing any energetic fields within them from escaping), salt lamps, increasing the number of plants in the home, and incorporating some of the practices listed at the end of this chapter. In extreme cases, people even refer to cell tower maps in order to move to safer, less "buzzy" areas, where they can put more distance between themselves and the power sources in order to feel more comfortable in their own skin.

With our escalating reliance on and close proximity to electronics—in our homes, in our offices, on our person—exposure to EMFs and their possible harm to human health have increasingly been debated by many scientists who are interested in whether the frequencies emitted by our toys may be affecting us in unseen ways. In 2011, the World Health Organization (WHO), after conducting a host of epidemiological studies, found evidence to support the theory that increased cell phone use correlates to various brain cancers and tumors, though it's still unclear just how much exposure is needed to create such outcomes. As a result, WHO classified radio-frequency electromagnetic fields as possibly carcinogenic to humans, noting an increased risk for glioma, a malignant brain cancer, in relation to cell phone use.[10]

Your handheld devices use radio frequency radiation to transmit signals to other phones—as well as to electronic devices like your computers, tablets, and watches. But your cell phone isn't just a tool to make phone calls anymore. They have evolved into smartphones, devices that perform as mini computers, typically with a touchscreen interface, internet access, and an operating system capable of running downloaded applications. These increased capabilities mean that we rely on our handheld devices more than ever, and that increased exposure brings additional danger. Non-ionizing radiation, which cell phones give off, has been thought to be safe because by definition it shouldn't be able to shift the structure of the molecules in our bodies. But a 2018 study conducted by the National Toxicology Program tested the effects of prolonged exposure to 2G and 3G radiation (not the 4G you are using at the time of this publication, nor the impending 5G that you will be exposed to very shortly) on rats and found clear evidence linking it to heart tumors. In

10 International Agency for Research on Cancer, "IARC Classifies Radiofrequency Electromagnetic Fields as Possibly Carcinogenic to Humans," May 31, 2011, https://www.iarc.fr/wp-content/uploads/2018/07/pr208_E.pdf.

other words, the radiation your cell phone emits may very well be on par with the radiation X-rays give off.

Remember when we were talking about free radicals and antioxidants in Chapter One? Free radicals are oxygen-containing molecules with an uneven number of electrons. Not all free radicals are bad or harmful; the body needs a certain amount to maintain health. It's just when they're produced in excess quantities that we should be concerned. That's where antioxidants come in, another superpower of shungite.

Antioxidants have the ability to donate electrons to free radicals in order to make them less reactive without making themselves unstable; shungite's reputably one of the most powerful free radical–fighting antioxidants. If there's an imbalance between free radicals and antioxidants in the body, this is called oxidative stress. When the body is exposed to harmful factors—radiation, pollution, secondhand smoke, certain pesticides and cleaners—the number of free radicals in the body multiplies, weakening the body's systems.

WAYS TO MAKE YOUR CELL PHONE EMIT LESS EMFS

- Turn off Bluetooth

- Turn off Wi-Fi

- Turn off GPS

- Turn off any app that asks to know your location

That means that sitting in close proximity to your phone, your computer, or anything with a Wi-Fi connection is adding regularly to the oxidative stress your body is under. Repeated studies show that EMFs given off by Wi-Fi are comparable to microwave EMFs,[11] causing oxidative stress, sperm/testicular damage, neuropsychiatric effects including shifts in electro-encephalogram (EEG, used to monitor electrical activity in the brain) readings, apoptosis (the death of cells), cellular DNA damage, endocrine changes, and calcium overload.

There's also evidence that non-ionizing radiation can mutate and fragment the DNA in our cells, specifically affecting calcium levels. Calcium is the most abundant mineral in the human body. And while we usually think of calcium as necessary to strengthen our bones and teeth, aka our skeletal structure, it's also needed for cell signaling, regulating enzyme and protein functions, muscle contraction, blood clotting, nerve function, cell growth, learning, and memory. Think of calcium as the body's chemical messenger.

To be clear, EMFs affect anything with DNA (including plants, animals, and insects). But where they do the most harm is in our voltage-gated calcium channels, or chambers within our cell membranes that allow calcium from outside the cell to move inside the cell. The cells in our bodies have evolved to regulate calcium levels. Exposure to EMFs increases calcium levels inside cells. Too much calcium in our cells creates

11   Martin L. Pall, "Wi-Fi Is an Important Threat to Human Health," *Environmental Research* 164 (March 2018): 405–416, https://www.sciencedirect.com/science/article/pii/S0013935118300355; Elfide Gizem Kıvrak et al., "Effects of Electro-magnetic Fields Exposure on the Antioxidant Defense System," *Journal of Microscopy and Ultrastructure* 5, no. 4 (2017): 167–176, https://www.ncbi.nlm.nih.gov/pmc/articles/PMC6025786.

oxidative stress, disrupting the information sent between synapses.

The brain, heart, and reproductive organs have the highest concentrations of calcium in the body and are the organs affected most by EMF exposure. Is it any wonder that, since the World Wide Web became publicly available in 1991, there has been unprecedented growth in chronic diseases related to the three areas? Brown University researcher Richard Lear, in his paper "The Root Cause in the Dramatic Rise of Chronic Disease," found that within a generation, there has been a huge uptick in diseases and disorders like autism (2,094%), Alzheimer's (299%), chronic obstructive pulmonary disease/COPD (148%), diabetes (305%), sleep apnea (430%), celiac disease (1,111%), ADHD (819%), asthma (142%), depression (280%), bipolar disease in youth (10,833%), osteoarthritis (449%), lupus (787%), inflammatory bowel disease/IBD (120%), chronic fatigue syndrome (11,027%), fibromyalgia (7,727%), multiple sclerosis (117%), and hypothyroidism (702%).[12] Is it coincidence that these are all extreme manifestations of electrohypersensitivity symptoms?

OKAY, SO WHAT DOES THIS ALL HAVE TO DO WITH SHUNGITE?

There is no doubt that we live among more electromagnetic fields now than ever. And while it may seem like there is

---

12   Richard Lear, "The Root Cause in the Dramatic Rise of Chronic Disease," Dramatic Rise in Chronic Disease Project, May 2016, https://www.researchgate.net/publication/303673576.

no escaping their deleterious effects, this is where shungite comes in.

Research has shown that shungite neutralizes the effects of electromagnetic radiation and weakens the effects of EMFs on the human body. The excitable energy of EMFs create or exacerbate anxiety. For those of us already prone to anxiety, who experience electrohypersensitivity, or who are in spaces—our homes, our office, or the city or town we live in—where there are high levels of EMFs, shungite works double-time to counterbalance active energy both outside and within ourselves.

The cage-like geometric lattice of shungite's fullerene structure is what enables EMF absorption, shielding the human body from the harmful radiation; its design is what attracts and traps those harmful excess free radicals we mentioned earlier as well.

If you have an EMF meter to read the amount of radiation you're exposed to in your home, here is a test you can conduct. Read the meter for total radiation in different areas of your home: in your bedroom, in an area of your house that has multiple electronics and/or appliances, and near your phone, taking note of the number in each area. Next, take a second reading, but this time, when you take your measurements from the same exact places you stood for the first readings, place a piece of shungite in each area or hold it near the meter. Then compare your findings. You'll be surprised at the difference it makes.

HOW TO USE SHUNGITE TO PROTECT YOURSELF AGAINST EMFS

On top of the above-mentioned practices, shungite is the simplest, most cost-effective way to protect yourself from damaging EMFs. All you have to do is place the mineral in strategic areas to let it work its magic. Just set it and forget it. Some of the most effective ways to place shungite around your home for your protection are:

- Alongside fully loaded power strips or anywhere lots of electrical wires commingle. *Recommended piece*: pyramid or generator

- Create a protective force field in a room that has many electrical appliances by placing one piece in each corner of the room. *Recommended piece*: cubes

- Carry a small piece in your pocket to keep yourself protected from EMFs or help curb anxiety at all times. *Recommended piece*: tumbled or raw pieces

- Keep a piece next to or under your bed to help with any sleep issues or insomnia. *Recommended piece*: pyramids

- Place next to Wi-Fi router or Ethernet cable. *Recommended piece*: pyramid or generator

- Place on the back of your cell phone. *Recommended piece*: There are small, flat pieces you can obtain that come with an adhesive material in order to attach to your phone

TIPS TO PROTECT YOURSELF AND YOUR HOME

- Switch to Ethernet internet instead of Wi-Fi: Ethernet is actually faster

- Unplug Wi-Fi from the wall at night

- Turn off your cell phone at night or put it on airplane mode

- Don't sleep with your cell phone in your room at night

- Remove all electrical devices from your sleeping area

- Turn off all circuits at night from the circuit breaker

- Reduce the amount of metal you're exposed to as metal is a conductor; radiation is attracted to metal and water

- Set a piece next to your computer or in a prominent place at your workstation. *Recommended piece*: Any piece will do, but pyramids and generators will be most effective

- Wear as jewelry to make your shungite work double-time as both protection and fashionable accessory. A range of necklaces, bracelets, rings, and earrings are available. *Necklace recommendation*: Get a pendant on a chain long enough that the shungite rests directly in front of the heart for maximum protection.

We have no idea all the ways technology will advance in the future, but if the past is any indication, it will continue to try to make our lives easier, testing the limits of what humans are capable of. With more advances will come even more EMFs, so placing shungite in some of the "hot spots" in your home is a natural yet effective way to reduce the dangerous effects of EMFs wreaking havoc on your DNA and deteriorating the energy systems embedded within us all. We'll take a closer look at how both EMFs and trauma affect our energy in the next chapters.

CHAPTER 5

The Aura

Your aura is the energy field that surrounds your body; it can extend from a few inches to several feet in front of you. Functioning as both a protective sheath and an "informer"— the means in which a person is able to receive intuitive information outside of themselves—it's both our connection and translator to the world around us, our own personal magnetic field that mimics the function and shape of the earth's.

This layer of protection was first measured scientifically by Harold Burr in his Yale laboratory in the 1930s, which he dubbed the *biofield*. Burr discovered that all living things were molded and controlled by electromagnetic properties, which he believed to be the organizing principle of all living tissue in all living things: humans, plants, and animals.[13]

We'd been referring to the aura long before science recognized it. This etheric body is described in numerous religions (Judaism, Christianity, Hinduism) and healing traditions

---

13   Ronald E. Matthews, "Harold Burr's Biofields Measuring the Electromagnetics of Life," *Bioelectromagnetic and Subtle Energy Medicine* 18, no. 2 (2007): 55–61, https://journals.sfu.ca/seemj/index.php/seemj/article/view/401.

(Chinese medicine, Ayurveda, qigong, yoga), and it surrounds and permeates all living systems; it's even depicted in religious art, surrounding Jesus and other saintly beings. It took a few millennia for science to catch up to what ancient teachings have preached.

Our aura isn't something we are given; it's not something we discover later in life. It's something we're born with, something necessary for life. Our aura carries spatial information that tells our fetal selves how to unfold in the womb and then, once on Earth, how our lives will develop—with all of our talents and quirks—out in the world. It's our data map on how we grow and take care of ourselves as adults.

The aura is one of two primary electrical systems in the body. We can think of the electrical systems of the human body as functioning similarly to AC/DC electricity. While the electric currents of the brain, heart, and muscles give off alternating on/off signals (like the alternating charges of AC), the aura's current is continuous; it's always on and flowing (like the energy of the earth: DC). The strength of the aura is determined by our level of consciousness, physical health, lifestyle, and surrounding environment. If there is a shift in any of these areas—be it positive or negative—the strength of our aura also shifts.

Without any deliberate effort, your energy is in constant interaction with the energy and matter that exists around you at all times. We're regularly monitoring and regulated by each other's biology, emotional states, and states of consciousness. Have you ever walked into a room or meeting while others were in an argument or heated debate? No one had to tell you that you probably walked in at the wrong time—you could just sense it. Your aura is what enables you to read both people and a space; it's your extrasensory perception. There may not be a logical reason that the mind can pinpoint to explain your feelings about being in a certain place, but your aura is perpetually picking up on the energetic information around you to help you make decisions, whether you're about to move into a new home, accept a job offer, or say yes to a date.

Noticing the energy around you helps you to experience a feeling of interconnectedness. When we feel connected, everything feels right, like we're in the right place or made the right decision. We feel in flow with the world around us.

FIGURE EIGHTS: THE PATTERN OF ENERGY

Feeling connected isn't just about having a strong energetic relationship with ourselves or those around us. It's also about our link to nature, where we came from. Human beings are natural-made organisms. We came from the earth. We evolved from the one-cell prokaryotes to Homo sapiens that carry thirty trillion cells. So the fact that the pattern of our energy field is mimicked by so many other natural elements should seem, well, natural.

This pattern both moves through us and surrounds us. The central axis of the aura, known as the torus or toroidal field, flows into the head via the crown chakra and exits out the groin or root chakra, circulating around the human body; its center is the heart. If you were able to see this energy as it moves in and out of you, it looks like a figure eight or infinity loop, the primary pattern for life found everywhere in nature, such as the cross section of an apple or grapefruit, the dynamic of a tornado, the structure of an atom, and the magnetic field around the earth. And it also surrounds you and me.

In the Hindu tradition, the *sushumna* channel, regarded as the energetic superhighway that runs along the spinal cord, connects the seven major chakras, allowing communication between the vortexes as it moves energy and information between them. Two alternating channels, *ida nadi* and *pingala nadi*, start at the root chakra and weave around each chakra located in the body, culminating at the sixth chakra (since the seventh chakra hovers in space) in a figure-eight pattern that helps each chakra connected to these *nadis* to spin and function.

The first six chakras (we'll learn more about all seven of them in the next chapter) are predominantly governed by one of these forces: *ida nadi* starts on the left side of the root chakra and is regarded as yin, feminine energy, associated with the moon, water, night, and the emotions (chakras two, four, six); *pingala nadi* starts on the right side and is seen as yang, masculine energy, associated with the sun, fire, day, and activity (chakras one, three, five). Chakras one through six are influenced by the energetic weaving of *ida* and *pingala nadis* around them.

The figure eight is a symbol of constant processing. In the original Rider-Waite tarot deck, this shape appears on the Magician, Strength, and Two of Pentacles cards. It symbolizes a deep connection to the Self for each archetype pictured on their respective cards, a sign that each character has the ability to channel information and is extremely in tune with their intuition. It's the shape of the earth's magnetic field, the human biofield, and even EMF radiation.

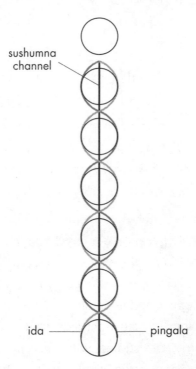

According to *Energy Medicine* author and founder Donna Eden, the aura is made up of energetic figure eights, the shape repeating itself over and over again around us. They dance around and move through us, offering us the ability to both channel information from outside of ourselves and interpret messages from the body—messages from within. The more figure eights there are weaving around you, the stronger your aura, the clearer your antennae. Though the aura's main purpose is to shield and protect us, the figure eights enable the aura to usher in external information for us to process and understand what's happening in the world around us at any given moment.

 AURA ENHANCER

Here's a simple exercise you can do with shungite to help strengthen your biofield. Holding a wand, tower, or any size or shape of shungite that you have, draw figure eights around you to strengthen your aura, boost your toroidal field, and create a stronger sheath of protection around you.

Draw them in front of you, to your left, to the right, behind you, on the soles of your feet, and above you over and over again for about 3 minutes. Continue for longer if you're feeling it.

The shungite will help to cleanse and purify your aura as you draw more figure eights to help strengthen it.

ENERGY FLOWS WHERE ATTENTION GOES

The strength of the auric field is directly affected by changes in our thoughts and moods. Our biofields harmonize and balance themselves via our thoughts and actions, specifically our repeated thoughts and actions. So if you're constantly second-guessing and questioning yourself, you not only will experience anxiety (which we'll talk more about in Chapter Seven) and indecisiveness but also will give off these unstable vibes.

Your aura will always be balanced, but that "balance" is determined by the energy you put out. No matter if you are perennially nervous or quite sure of yourself, your aura will exist in harmony with your thoughts. So if you're feeling confident, your aura will feel strong and expansive; if you're feeling anxious, it will contract.

This is why there are some people who seem to effortlessly captivate our attention, while others are unmemorable. Those who display a hypnotizing presence have strong, extended auras and give off a high vibration, while the auras of those who seem more vanilla shrink back and away from the world around them and give off a lower vibration.

Think back to a time when you had a crush on someone. When in close proximity to someone you're attracted to, you're acutely aware of exactly where they are in the room and how close they are in relation to you without necessarily needing to see or touch them. The hairs on your arms stand on end, your pulse quickens, your palms get sweaty, your heart races. All of your attention and energy focuses on the object of your affection. It's nothing physical that the body can touch that alerts you to their every move or the feeling that you get when you're near them; your aura picks up on the energetic information emanating from them, the frequencies their biofield puts out. The reason you were attracted to this person is because you liked the way their energy made you feel when you were around them. You dug their vibe. You were "picking up what they were putting down." Your energy was in conversation with theirs.

ENERGY EXCHANGE

We're constantly exchanging information with the world around us, taking information in and sending information out. One of the ways we do this is with our breath, a constant circular flow of receiving and releasing that feeds our body not only with the oxygen it requires but also with information needed to help us read a room.

Since breathing is a natural function of the body that occurs without us having to think about it, we often don't consider it. Take a few moments to close your eyes and note where in your body you feel the breath. If you're unsure how to notice or locate it, feel into where your physical body may move because of your breathing.

Often the place where we feel or notice our breath most is in the chest. Maybe you were aware of the breath in the higher regions of your chest on the front side of your body, but the longer you sat with your eyes closed, concentrating, the sensation may have dropped lower—into the lungs or rib-cage area. This is because when we turn off outside stimulation (or close our eyes), we're able to focus deeply on what we are doing: breathing.

Shallow breathing is an indicator of a contracted aura. If we're only breathing into the front side of the body, we're only fueling one-fourth of our innate protection and channeling system, ignoring 75 percent of our capacity to sense what's happening in the world around us. Seventy-five percent! If we're using that little of it, then what's the point of having this powerful, invisible sheath that helps us do so much?

The aura is meant to expand in all directions in order to be most effective. If you were to think of your aura as a bubble, and you were only breathing shallow breaths to the front side of the body, your aura would still fully surround you—it just would hug close to your body. Ideally, we want it to extend as far away from us as possible in all directions so that we can pick up more information and be more fully aware of our surroundings, comparable in size to Glinda the Good Witch's bubble in *The Wizard of Oz*.

Even in a weakened state, though, the aura remains whole. Whatever its size, however big or small it is in any given moment, it self-regulates. It still works in a condensed state; it just isn't as effective. This is where shungite comes in.

A weak aura can't discern what's good or bad energetically; it can't differentiate what's high vibe versus low; it can't be firm with its boundaries; it can't sense when things are off. Our success and happiness rely on our ability to choose what's right for us; when our aura is feeble, we can't choose things intentionally or intuitively. Research has shown that, when worn or carried, shungite is capable of expanding and strengthening the aura, doubling its size and range.

HOW FAR WILL SHUNGITE EXPAND YOUR AURA?

The distance the aura can extend with shungite is affected by the number of EMFs being emitted in the area you are in. Your aura will expand to great lengths if you're outdoors and away from laptops, cell phones, and Wi-Fi; it will still extend with shungite when these or other electronic devices are present—it just won't be as expansive.

Here's a fun experiment you can try to see the difference in the size of your aura with and without shungite, around electronics and outside:

What you need:

> » a partner

> » two aura markers (to mark where you make contact with the other person's aura); you can use mugs, seashells, books, deodorant—whatever you like!

> » pair of copper dowsing rods

Note: *Dowsing rods, or divining rods (shaped like the letter L), have been used over time to find underground water sources and buried treasure. The rods* *respond to unconscious electrical movements within our muscles, but in order to get an effective reading, the person holding the rods needs to be in a calm, relaxed state.*

1. Hold on to the shorter prongs of the dowsing rods while allowing the longer prongs to point away from you. Similar to a pendulum, you need to ask the rods questions to discover how they will move for a *no* answer versus how they will move for *yes*. You must do this each time you use the dowsing rods, whether you're using them to test the strength of your aura, test the strength of your shungite, make better-informed decisions about life, or search for lost valuables. While holding the rods, ask them: "Show me *yes*," and notice how they move, if they both sway in one direction or cross each other in the middle. Once you've got your *yes*, say, "Reset," and watch them come back to center. Then ask: "Show me *no*," and note what they do for a *no* response.

Note: *You can practice this test using both rods or just one. If you're trying to test both and you notice that one is moving a lot more than the other, conduct the test holding just the one dowsing rod in the hand in which you noticed more movement.*

2. Once you determine how your rods will move, stand about 6 feet away from the person whose aura you are testing, with the long prongs pointing straight out in front of you. Say to the dowsing rods: "Show me when I've made contact with [name]'s aura," and slowly begin to walk toward your partner. The dowsing rods will move in the direction of your *yes* when you've come in contact with your partner's aura. Place an aura marker on the ground where you stood when your dowsing rods moved.

3. Next, have your partner hold a piece of shungite to see how far their aura extends with the aura-strengthening mineral. This time allow more space between you and your partner, standing at least 10 to 12 feet away from them with the long prongs pointing straight out in front of you. Again, say to the dowsing rods: "Show me when I've made contact with [name]'s aura," and slowly begin to walk toward your partner. The dowsing rods will move in the direction of your *yes* when you've come in contact with your partner's aura. Place an aura marker on the ground where you stood when your dowsing rods moved.

4. Measure the distance between the two aura markers to see how much farther the shungite helped expand your partner's aura.

Try out this test inside your home or office, around your electronics, taking note of how close to the body your aura is when in the presence of many positive ions. Then try it outside to notice your aura's sphere where there are more negative ions present.

If you have multiple pieces of shungite of differing sizes, complete the test with all of them to discover their differing ranges. Engaging in this experiment will show you firsthand shungite's protective qualities, proving how rare and powerful this mineral is. Once you see it, you'll believe it.

THE PATH OF LEAST RESISTANCE

Here's the thing about energy: it flows along the path of least resistance. If it bumps up against a blockage or areas that are more stagnant, energy shifts its course in order to avoid conflict. It would much rather find a go-around than deal with confrontation. If traversed often enough, the path of least resistance becomes further and further carved out, eventually becoming the new normal, an update to our natural state.

When a moving body of water confronts a "blockage" in the form of a dam or boulder, it shifts course to try to get around it; over time, if the block is not removed, the water wears away at the earth and rock on its new path, carving out a new route, deepening its groove within the earth, making it that much harder to redirect its course when confronted with another block. If, while eating, we burn or scratch ourselves inside our mouths on the side we chew on, only then do we learn to chew our food on the other side to avoid the pain of irritating the favored side more. The brain of a recovering stroke patient learns to rewire itself in order to relay necessary information on how to communicate or respond to physical stimuli, allowing the survivor to regain the functions they lost from the damage the stroke caused the brain. Neurotransmitters create new road maps to different areas of the brain to take over functions that may no longer seem to compute with portions of the brain put permanently offline.

Confronted with a blockage, problem, or dead zone, the water, our mouths, and the brain each have to renegotiate their paths in order to be able to carry out their specific functions. Each has no other choice but to find new ways to operate. Our energy, on the other hand, will continue to follow the path of least resistance unless we come at it with an awareness to consciously shift its course. The difference is that the blocks our energy encounters are invitations to interpret them not as blocks, but as bridges that allow us to advance and grow into more evolved beings. Working with shungite, however, can help us navigate through our own personal blocks if we feel empowered to make significant changes in our life.

In order to rewire and strengthen your energy, carrying a piece of shungite in your pocket at all times or wearing it as jewelry can help protect you from negative energy from the people around you. At first, the shungite, like your aura, will act just as a protective sheath to help stop toxic energy from affecting you. But wearing or being exposed to shungite long enough will also help inspire you to rewire your own energy: from making more positive decisions; to weeding out any harmful habits, foods, or people from your life; to inspiring you to work on any parts of yourself that need more love and healing. Put simply, shungite can help you drastically transform yourself from the inside out.

To be clear, just having a piece of shungite on you won't automatically make you more aware or help you make better decisions the moment you place it in your pocket. Just as any interpersonal relationship evolves over time, so, too, does the one you have with this mineral. It will start to enhance your energy from the get-go, but in order for it to help revolutionize your life, you have to develop a connection to it.

Here is a DIY way to work with shungite on a daily basis that will aid in strengthening and expanding your biofield.

 AURA SPRAY

Use shungite to help cleanse your aura by creating your own spray to use after spending time around electronics, when you're feeling anxious, or just to give your biofield a boost.

What you need:

» 4–6 pieces of elite shungite 0.5–1.5 centimeters in diameter (**Note**: *Because of elite shungite's high carbon makeup, it's extremely powerful, so you won't need much, but the total number of pieces you use will depend on the size.*)

» 2- to 4-ounce small spray misting bottle

» distilled water

» small clear quartz crystals, to enhance (optional)

1. First, clean your shungite. Use filtered water to gently scrub away any black residue, mud, and other impurities with your hands or a brush. Do not use soap.

2. If your pieces of elite shungite are too big to fit in the bottle, gently press a few fragile pieces to break into smaller pieces. Because this is a spray, using the finer crumbs that may seem too small is completely acceptable—none of your shungite needs to go to waste.

3. Place 4–6 pieces of elite shungite in the bottle, along with the clear quartz crystals if also using.

4. Fill the bottle with distilled water.

5. Secure the cap on the bottle.

6. Spray on and around yourself for an instant aura boost.

Enhancing the energy around us will also help restore the energy within us. We'll take a deeper look at this—and ourselves—as we familiarize ourselves with the energy centers that exist within us and learn how their health affects our own physical, mental, and emotional well-being in the next chapter.

CHAPTER 6

The Chakras

All of our experiences shape who we become. The good, the bad, the ugly—each plays a role in molding us as individuals: positive reinforcement, the death of a loved one, being teased at school, being popular at school, not being able to afford the styles or labels fashionable at the time. Every single event that we live through affects not just our energy, but our entire way of being, whether we realize it or not. The energetic memory of each experience we've survived and our reaction to it is stored in our body. The saying "The issues are in our tissues" speaks to how the body holds on to emotional memories. Every single person on the planet has a completely unique emotional landscape that can trigger anxiety when met with experiences that fan the flames of our core wounds and elicit similar unpleasant reactions.

In Sanskrit, the word *chakra* translates to "wheel." Chakras are wheels of energy that flow within the body. The chakra system dates back to 1500–500 BC. It was first referenced in the Vedas, one of Hinduism's oldest known scriptures. It's believed that there are hundreds of small chakras in the body, but there are seven main energy centers located along the length of the spine. The placement of each varies from person to person. Some chakras may sit slightly off to the left or right of the vertebral column, but each has a specific energy that corresponds to our mental, emotional, and spiritual state and influences certain organs and physical features that lie within its energy field. If a chakra is blocked or out of balance, it can cause disharmony and discomfort, affecting us on a mental or emotional level. If the imbalance is left unchecked, the energetic blockage can accumulate, eventually causing physical issues and/or disease.

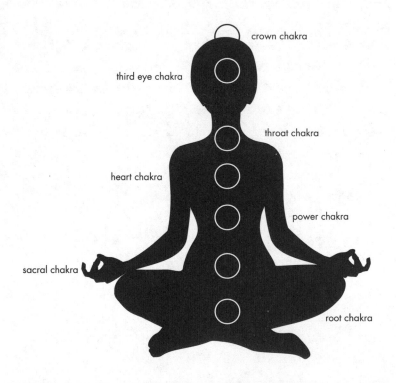

crown chakra

third eye chakra

throat chakra

heart chakra

power chakra

sacral chakra

root chakra

In the 1970s, Dr. Valerie Hunt discovered that the human body did, in fact, produce rapid electrical oscillations that correspond with the descriptions of the ancient texts that refer to the chakras. Hunt's studies showed that when the chakras are in balance, there is synchronicity between them; the energy of each flows properly on its own, allowing them to work cohesively together. But when chakras are blocked or operating less than optimally, they fall out of sync with the others, and the whole system is affected.

The growth and development of our chakras is strikingly similar to how our crystal friends came into being. Just as the location of igneous rock formation and the perfect swirl of mineral-forming elements determine what rock is formed, the location of our birth (in terms of astrology), the perfect swirl of our biological parents' DNA, and our living environment determine who we become, with all of our strengths and weaknesses. As we grow, outside elements—this time in the form of family, school, friends, and even strangers—reshape our personality as we start to find ourselves and our way in the world, comparable to how sedimentary rocks are formed under the thumb of nature's elements. The wisdom that comes with age allows us to look back on our lives to see not only where we can work to grow mentally, emotionally, or spiritually, but also what needs healing, what needs to be embraced, how we might be able to look at different events from our lives and see their effects on us, what patterns or habits we can let go of, and how we can transform ourselves from the inside out. Similar to the literal pressure a rock withstands that reorganizes its internal structure to make a metamorphic rock more resistant, when the pressures of life are thrust upon us, we're forced into our own metamorphosis, fortifying our resiliency.

The chakras hold the blueprints that map out our strengths, our weaknesses, and our suffering. They communicate with each other, sharing energetic information in order to understand and interpret how the entire energy system can work collectively to keep us healthy and safe. If we experience pain or distress, energy is rushed in from other areas of the body to help. This is how our energy centers—and all systems of the body—function when thrown into fight or flight. When we suddenly find ourselves in scary, uncomfortable, or compromised circumstances, the human body by design is programmed to direct all its energy into getting out of sticky situations—alive. Think of it as a safety feature. If this reaction is prolonged or consistently triggered, energy can get stuck flowing in one direction to help facilitate healing, creating new blockages in the areas the body has been pulling the energy from.

Since they're constantly communicating and exchanging energy, one chakra out of whack can throw off the energy of any or all of the other chakras, as well as the aura, because the two energy systems are inextricably linked. This is why it's important to understand how each chakra works, and how the strength or weakness of one can influence the strength or weakness of them all.

Here we'll take a look at all seven chakras; where each is located; their energetic properties; the types of experiences that could block, hinder, or facilitate growth in each area; and how shungite's unique healing qualities can help us achieve balance in each energy center.

THE SELF AND DIVINE

I'll be using the terms Self and Divine in this chapter.

The **Self** refers to our highest, most pure self, the essence of who we are, the part of our being that already knows all the answers, whom we spend most of our lives trying to connect and unite with.

Divine is a word I've chosen to describe the sacred force that is responsible for all life on this planet. It is the force that causes the grass to grow, the wind to blow. It's the whispers that echo through our body and our being that urge us to take risks, say no to anything that isn't in our highest good, and say yes to everything that is. If the term *Divine* doesn't work or feel right to you, swap it out for one that does: Source, Creator, God, Goddess, Life Force, Rita, your word if you have one, or something completely different that speaks to you. Your energy speaks differently from mine. Use the term that feels most aligned for you.

FIRST CHAKRA • ROOT CHAKRA • MULADHARA

Location: the base of the spine near the perineum, the space between the sex organs

Association: survival, safety, and security; being provided for; feeling "at home" or grounded within one's self; trust; shelter, protection, our basic needs

Governs: the sacrococcygeal/sacral plexus; anus, rectum; immune system; hips, legs, knees, ankles, feet

The formation of the first chakra begins when we are still in the womb. It holds the energy of our origin story—not just how we were conceived, but the energy of the home we're born into. Everyone has different needs to feel safe and provided for; these needs are defined by whatever love and care we did or didn't receive from one, both, or any of our caregivers.

Experiences that happen in early childhood have a lasting impact on our first chakra that affects what we must work on shifting and healing as adults.

Here is a list of situations that can cause this chakra to be closed off or in need of attention and strengthening:

• Living in a home where a caregiver was verbally or physically abusive

• Living in a home where a caregiver was often absent or unable to be fully present and spend time with you

- Feeling abandoned by your family or caregivers

- Living in a home that didn't have a lot of money or where clothes and food (basic human needs) were hard to come by

- Living in an unsafe area or neighborhood

- Living in an area where you or your family were not accepted

- Moving around a lot

- Feeling a strong distaste or hate for the values your caregivers modeled and tried to instill you

The conditions and energy of our home life and living situations affect us just as much as the food we consume, if not more so. Being cared for, feeling loved, and having a roof over our head are basic human needs. If something gets in the way of these needs, it will affect our feelings of safety and our survival skills in the future.

Shungite can help us find the courage to sit with ourselves to observe our past in relation to our root chakra and the emotions associated with what we've been through. It can help us ground our energy by calming the frequencies of the upper chakras, neutralizing any EMFs nearby, and helping stabilize blood pressure to make it feel easier and less daunting to focus our attention inward to start to heal our relationship to our past. Shungite can help us transform our foundation into a robust source of strength, something we can come back to and rely on rather than run away from. It can help invite a sense of calm for us to harmonize and rebalance our root chakra energy.

USING SHUNGITE TO SUPPORT YOUR ROOT CHAKRA

One of the simplest, easiest ways to ground first chakra energy is to keep tumbled pieces of shungite to the touch or added pressure, so that they're as close as physically possible to your root chakra during your day. Elite pieces are too fragile and will crumble to the touch or added pressure, so using Petrovsky or black shungite will be your cleanest, best bet. Before placing in your pocket, sit with the piece(s) you will be carrying with you and set an intention for your first chakra.

Examples of affirmations or intentions for the root chakra:

- I am grounded
- I am safe
- I have all I need
- My needs are taken care of

For a more interactive way to ground root chakra energy, meditate holding a sphere or harmonizer in each hand. I recommend using the shungite/steatite combination as the yin and yang energies noticeably calm your energy and naturally invite in more stillness than using two identical pieces of shungite.

 SQUARE GRID

The best grid shape for enhancing the energy of the root chakra is a square. The shape of a square or a cube, with its six evenly shaped faces (four sides, top, and bottom), helps promote and maintain stability.

1. If you only have one piece of shungite, make it the centerpiece of your square gird and surround it with four other crystals, one in each corner, to amplify stable shungite energy.

2. If you have four cube pieces, create a square with them, feeling out the distance between them that feels harmonious and balanced to you.

Another powerful way to use a grid to help balance and strengthen your root chakra is becoming a part of the grid yourself.

1. Sit with four cubes of shungite surrounding you.

2. If you have harmonizers, hold them in your hands as well.

3. Meditate for 5–10 minutes on your own or using the grounding cord meditation described below.

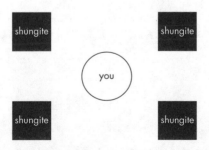

GROUNDING CORD MEDITATION

This is one of my favorite, most grounding meditation practices. You will want to hold two pieces of shungite, preferably the same size and shape, in either hand.

1. Set a timer for your desired meditation time.

2. Come to a comfortable seat, rooting your tailbone down toward the earth, the crown of your head extending upward toward the sky.

3. Close your eyes and let your breath come naturally, paying attention to your breathing for a few moments—where you feel it move within you, the lengths of your breaths.

4. Start to bring your awareness to your tailbone, the base of your spine.

5. Imagine a cord growing out of your tailbone, lengthening and lowering down into the earth. Watch for a few breaths as it continues to move downward, further and further toward the center of the earth.

6. On an inhale, envision drawing energy up the cord back into your body; as you exhale, send the energy back down the cord.

7. Continue to visualize this energetic conversation you're having with the earth with each breath, drawing earth energy up and into yourself via your grounding cord with each inhale, releasing energy back down the cord and into the earth with each exhale.

8. Repeat until your timer goes off.

SECOND CHAKRA • SACRAL CHAKRA • SVADHISTHANA

Location: lower belly, between the pelvic floor and navel

Association: creativity, sexuality, money, how we relate to others: family, friends, partners, coworkers

Governs: the reproductive and urinary organs and systems, large intestine, appendix, lower back/sacrum

The second chakra is perhaps the most complicated and complex energy center in the human body. Known as "the dwelling place of the Self," this is the home of our personality, all the unique quirks that make us who we are. Ruling over our reproductive organs, the sacral chakra also governs sexuality and creativity. Ideas are born from this chakra, giving birth to something, not necessarily just babies, but our identity—this is where ideas are made manifest. It's from this energy center that we are imbued with the urge to create.

Creativity emerges from all of us in different ways. It's not necessarily about being artistic but the eyes through which we see the world, the ways we attempt to color our own existence. It can come through as dancing or playing sports, how we dress, home decor, the way we prepare our meals, or the way we style our hair. The second chakra is the seat of our desires, the things we want or the things we yearn for that give us and our lives meaning. Creative energy is just an outward expression of what we're drawn to.

Experiences that can cause the second chakra to be closed off or in need of attention and strengthening:

- Being teased at school for something you did, said, or wore

- A caregiver making a remark that caused you to feel bad or ashamed about something you did

- A caregiver not taking your creative attempts or pursuits seriously, putting you down, not believing the thing you wanted to do would be able to support you

- A caregiver forcing you to pursue a hobby that they chose for you without taking your own desires into account

- Sexual trauma or abuse

- Feeling controlled by others, or a fear of losing control

- Betrayal

When this energy center is blocked or out of balance, it's hard for us to stay true to ourselves. Our experiences mold us into the people we become, directly affecting both our strengths and our weaknesses. The need to feel liked and accepted is one of the most important basic human desires. When there is a lack of connection to the Self, or if our desires aren't met or our ideas aren't accepted, we learn to hide the parts of ourselves that elicit disappointment, concern, or scolding, or that start disagreements, even if it's something that makes our hearts sing. Because we want to feel praised and accepted, we learn to hold back the parts of ourselves that don't receive praise or acceptance, second-guessing our urges if they're not socially adequate.

For anyone who has experienced trauma, the mind and body, meant to work together, sometimes have differing ideas of how to stay safe. Dissociation is a common coping method among survivors of abuse. Turning off what we feel or pretending we're somewhere more pleasant instead of being present for the pain are ways we disconnect from the full impact of the trauma to help cope with an otherwise unbearable experience. If we detach from ourselves, even as a means of protection, it's impossible to have a strong sense of Self.

Someone with a strong sense of Self, a strong second chakra, will stand up for their Self. They trust their urges and desires and follow through with them. It's not that they don't care what people think, it's just that they trust themselves over the ideas and advice of others. If there have been trauma or negative experiences in relation to discovering and expressing the Self, healing work is necessary to reestablish the strength of this energy center.

Because of shungite's ability to absorb negative energy, it is an extremely powerful aid that allows us to transform our relationship with ourselves and our sacral chakra by allowing us to identify our distorted thoughts and feelings. It's only after we recognize them and call them out that we can start to let them go to create space for new, more loving and accepting beliefs to trickle in.

USING SHUNGITE TO SUPPORT YOUR SACRAL CHAKRA

Lying down and resting a piece of shungite on your sacral chakra is one of the simplest, easiest ways to ground second chakra energy. Since we spend most of the day sitting or moving around, though, carrying a tumbled piece or two via a fanny pack will help you keep the mineral as close to your sacral chakra as possible no matter what you do throughout your day. Before you start wearing them, set an intention to help you start to strengthen your second chakra.

Examples of affirmations or intentions for the sacral chakra:

- I love who I am
- I attract people in my life who love and appreciate me
- I have great ideas
- People love me for who I am
- My creativity is as unique as I am

 ## SACRAL CHAKRA FIGURE EIGHTS

Wearing the fanny pack in which you've placed some shungite as suggested above, stand with your feet about hips distance apart. Start to draw figure eights with your hips to help build the energy of your second chakra and shake free any stagnant or stuck energy that may be causing a blockage or standing in the way of your creativity, sexual energy, or any of your likes and loves that you've felt too scared to share or experience. Turn on one of your favorite high-energy songs and shake out whatever has been standing in your way.

 SPIRAL GRID

One of the most potent grid shapes to inspire creativity and help you connect to your own unique energy is a spiral grid. The spiral is a sacred shape that is a metaphor for life: we will never be in the same place in our lives twice because we are constantly growing, changing, and evolving. Even if we never leave the contentment of our comfort zones, our cells are still reproducing and dying off, constantly replacing each other so that even moment to moment we are never the same.

1. Place a pyramid or tower of shungite in the center.

2. Build outward with other crystals—or more shungite—in a spiral formation.

3. Write your intention on a piece of paper, fold it up, and place it under the center stone.

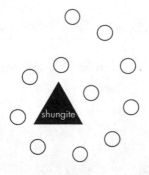

THIRD CHAKRA • POWER CHAKRA • MANIPURA

Location: solar plexus; the space between the navel and the heart, around the lower ribs

Association: the seat of our drive, self-confidence, courage, determination, self-esteem, empowerment, and boundaries

Governs: the adrenals (which sit atop the kidneys and produce hormones that help regulate your metabolism, immune system, blood pressure, response to stress, and other essential functions), kidneys, digestive system, stomach, liver, pancreas, spleen, lumbar spine

The third chakra is the source of our drive, endurance, and determination. It's from this space that we find the courage to do something new, take risks, and respect ourselves enough to establish boundaries with coworkers, partners, and family members. This energy is meant to push us forward, but if blocked or weak it can end up holding us back. It's the fire within us, our vitality.

If we struggle to tend our fire, we're more apt to feel disconnected from our power. Detachment from this energy center translates into difficulties in finding the will or energy to initiate anything, from conversations with friends and loved ones to implementing new ideas we've had that could improve our lives. We're afraid to take the reins, steer the ship, stand out. Instead of feeling powerful, we feel power*less*, more prone to anxiety, self-doubt, or self-criticism.

The pendulum of imbalance swings both ways, though. When there is excess fire or energy hovering around the power chakra, it can present itself in someone overrun by ego or narcissism, which can make them more apt to manipulate or exert their power over others in order to satisfy their own needs and get what they want.

In its purest state, the third chakra is about connecting to our agency and potential, integrating our personal power into different aspects of the Self, of life, which should enhance, empower, and strengthen not just ourselves but everyone around us. Misuse of power is corruption, using our faculties at the expense of others. Power used properly is purifying and focused on what's highest and best for all beings.

Any blockages that we may have felt surrounding our second chakra inform how we show up in the third chakra: it's hard to feel confident or have a strong self-esteem if we've been sacrificing our needs and urges in order to satisfy others, gain approval, and keep the peace. If we're made to feel bad about certain aspects of ourselves or hold ourselves back long enough, shame stops us dead in our tracks from achieving any growth or self-acceptance, which keeps us from ever even touching our power.

Shame is one of the strongest emotions humans experience; it has a direct correlation to both the second and third chakras. Nationally renowned psychiatrist, physician, researcher, spiritual teacher, and lecturer David R. Hawkins mapped out the energy fields of human emotions. His "Map of Consciousness" shows the spectrum of emotions from the lowest frequency (shame) to the highest (enlightenment), illustrating shame as the force most destructive to our emotional and psychological health. It drains us of our energy, poisons our dreams of possibility, paralyzes us from taking action in our own lives, and creates anxiety, making us second-guess ourselves in both our thoughts and our actions, which translates to a lack of self-confidence or belief in ourselves and what we're capable of.

If we don't believe in our potential and abilities, the sovereignty of our power chakra will never be strong, and we'll lack the determination and drive to follow through on our dreams and what's important to us.

Experiences that can cause the third chakra to be closed off or in need of attention and strengthening:

- Being shut down, ignored, or made to feel like a failure after a display of courage

- Fear of rejection

- Criticism

- Anxiety over physical appearance

- Fear of being misunderstood

When the power chakra is blocked or out of balance, anxiety, worry, nervousness, self-consciousness, or lack of drive or willpower are likely familiar experiences, sometimes even the norm.

Working with shungite can help strengthen our will and determination. Because of its harmonizing qualities, shungite can help balance an underactive or overactive third chakra to help us discover and stand tall in our own power. Plus, since the third chakra governs the immune system and shungite has demonstrative powers to strengthen immunity, it is a great crystal to work with to help alchemize your strength from the inside out.

USING SHUNGITE TO SUPPORT YOUR POWER CHAKRA

To help you connect more directly with your power, find the Wonder Woman stance: stand with your feet wider than your hips, hands in fists resting on hips—while holding a harmonizer in either hand. You have to take up space in order to take this stance, which not only helps boost self-confidence and build self-esteem, but also helps strengthen and expand the aura.

Examples of affirmations or intentions for the power chakra:

- I am confident
- I am powerful
- I am strong
- I have strong boundaries
- I love and accept myself

 THREE-DIMENSIONAL BREATHING

This exercise can be done while in the Wonder Woman stance described above or seated comfortably. Since the third chakra lies roughly at the base of the diaphragm, you can use your breath to help you connect to your personal power. Hold a harmonizer or sphere in either hand. If you choose to sit while practicing this, let the backs of your hands rest about mid-thigh so that the elbows are bent, resting close to the body.

1. With your eyes closed, take a few breaths on your own, allowing the breath to come as it will. Notice yourself in relation to the space around you, notice how you're feeling in this moment, notice where you feel your breath.

2. Next, start to breathe into the front and back of the chest at once, breathing toward both the space in front of you and the space behind you. Breathe like this for 1–3 minutes. Take note of any shifts in your posture.

3. Shift your awareness to the sides of your body and begin to breathe more fully to the left and right as if you were trying to breathe your rib cage toward your arm-pits. Breathe like this for 1–3 minutes. Take note of any shifts in your posture.

4. Put all of it together, breathing toward the front and back of the chest, as well as either side. Breathe like this for 1–3 minutes or longer. Notice how breathing in all directions feels in relation to the previous steps. Notice how it feels to breathe more fully, both within and with-out, and directly into the solar plexus. Take note of any shifts in your awareness, as well as whether you sense more or less than when you began this exercise.

STAR GRID

One of the most powerful grids you can make to help boost self-confidence and self-esteem and help strengthen and maintain your personal power is a closed star grid.

1. Place a large piece of shungite (a pyramid, sphere, or tower are best, but any piece will work) in the middle.

2. Place five other large crystals (they can all be shungite, or whatever you have) around your centerpiece to create a star shape.

3. Connect the centerpiece to the point with smaller crystals so it looks like five lines are radiating from the center.

4. Close the circle up by adding smaller crystals in between the end points to amplify the energy.

5. Write your intention on a piece of paper, fold it up, and place it under the center stone.

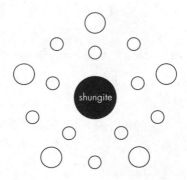

FOURTH CHAKRA • HEART CHAKRA • ANAHATA

Location: the heart

Association: love, hate, grief, anger, resentment, bitterness, forgiveness, and compassion

Governs: the heart, lungs, circulatory system, thymus gland, thoracic spine, arms, hands; our connection to other beings

The heart is our emotional center, the most powerful source of electromagnetic energy in the human body. It produces the largest rhythmic electromagnetic field of any of the body's organs. It's also where the energies of the upper chakras and lower chakras meet, the bridge between our inner and outer worlds, the connector of the Self and Divine. This is the first chakra of the main chakra system where energy rises up and out.

Where the previous three chakras define who you are and help you remain connected to yourself, the heart chakra looks to connect the Self outward to others. It's from the heart that we give and receive information in a circular, rhythmic cycle. The lungs surround the heart, taking in oxygen and information from the world around us when we inhale, releasing carbon dioxide (food for the trees) and information (that other people's auras pick up on) with the exhale; it's our emotional processor, allowing us to connect to the world around us emotionally and energetically.

Experiences that can cause this chakra to be closed off or in need of attention and strengthening:

- Not receiving the love you needed or desired as an infant, child, and/or adolescent

- Not receiving the love you feel you deserve as an adult

- The death of someone meaningful to you

- Romantic breakups

- Friend breakups

- Feeling let down by a parent or caregiver

- Ghosting (i.e., ending a relationship by ceasing all contact and communication with a friend or partner without ever providing an explanation or explicitly saying the relationship is over)

Feelings of insecurity that enter into our consciousness and our energy via the first three chakras express themselves here. All humans strive for acceptance and love; there are no two greater forces. If we don't feel accepted—by others or, more importantly, by ourselves—the pain that comes with rejection motivates us to harden around the heart, erect (imaginary) walls, and develop a thicker skin for protection and self-preservation.

Shungite is a powerful mineral to work with to help soften the armor around the heart to transform our patterns and rewire the energy that flows through our emotional center, allowing us to break free from the pain of our past, find more compassion for and acceptance of ourselves, and open up to both give and receive more love. The fourth chakra responds to shungite similarly to the way our aura does: expanding the energy center and neutralizing the effects of negative emotions on the heart while at the same time shielding it from other outside adverse forces.

USING SHUNGITE TO SUPPORT YOUR HEART CHAKRA

Shungite helps the heart center discern what energy comes in and what is released from us, so it can be quite effective in letting go of emotions that have hardened our heart or perhaps closed us off to love, inviting in more compassion for ourselves and others, even the ones who have caused us pain.

Examples of affirmations or intentions for the heart chakra:

- I am worthy of love

- I forgive myself

- I have compassion for all beings

- I love myself unconditionally

- My emotions are my teachers

 PINK LIGHT BUBBLE MEDITATION

Practice the following meditation with a harmonizer or sphere in either hand to help boost and protect the power of your heart.

1. Come to a nice, tall, comfortable seat.

2. Close your eyes and begin to notice your breath.

3. Imagine yourself sitting in a bubble, your entire body completely surrounded.

4. Sitting in the bubble, start to bring your awareness to your heart space.

5. In the middle of your heart, start to notice a small pink light begin to emerge.

6. Watch the pink light start to grow bigger and stronger as you breathe into it with each breath, expanding it in all directions.

7. Continue to expand the pink light with each breath until your heart is completely full of this light.

8. Feel your heart full of this light, your light, your love, your energy, your life force.

9. Begin to shoot that pink light from your heart into the bubble.

10. Continue to visualize that pink light shooting out from your heart and into the bubble until you are completely surrounded, completely engulfed in the pink light.

11. In this bubble, surrounded by your light, your love, your energy, your life force, you are completely protected. No one else's energy can penetrate the bubble. No one else's energy can harm you or affect you. Any energy that tries to come into your field will bounce off your bubble. You are safe. You are protected. You are

protected by your own light, your own love, your own energy, your own life force.

12. Sit here a few moments, basking in your energy field, allowing it to both protect you and fuel you. When you are ready, slowly begin to open your eyes.

 FIGURE EIGHT GRID

Creating a crystal grid in the form of a figure eight can help boost the energy of your heart chakra as it mimics the shape of the toroidal field, energy flowing in and out of the heart center.

1. Place a large piece of shungite (a pyramid, sphere, or tower are best, but any piece will work) in the middle.

2. Using any other crystals you have, create the infinity loop around the center stone, mimicking the shape of our toroidal field.

3. Write your intention on a piece of paper, fold it up, and place it under the center stone.

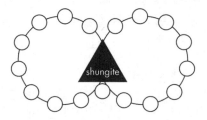

FIFTH CHAKRA • THROAT CHAKRA • VISHUDDHA

Location: base of the throat

Association: communication, self-expression, creative expression, speaking your truth, channel for Divine wisdom to speak through you

Governs: the throat, thyroid gland (which secretes the necessary hormones for all the cells in your body to function healthily and regulates metabolism), parathyroid (governs calcium absorption and release in the body), cervical spine

The throat is believed to be the body's gatekeeper, allowing in food and air substances that literally feed us what we need for physical survival and nourishment. It's also what enables us to communicate with others using our voice. The fifth chakra is where we both transmit and receive information, the place where consciousness—an awareness of our thoughts, feelings, sensations, and external surroundings and our interpretations of them—extends outside us.

Communication is one of the most integral aspects of this energy center. It's the great connector. It's how and why we form relationships with others: we like or agree with what the people we invite into our life have to say; we avoid those who don't share our values. Conversation is how we specify our values and often how we learn what is important to others, but the throat chakra's role in communication extends beyond what we say out loud.

Every living thing gives off a vibration. It's through vibration that information is transmitted and received. It can be through the intonation and resonance of our voice; it can be through the rhythmic pulsations of the neurotransmitters that communicate messages to the brain. It's the rhythm of energy that we pick up on when we enter a room and understand that something good or uncomfortable just happened.

All of our chakras give off a vibration. The vibrations of the lower chakras are fainter, but as we travel up the spine, their rhythms become more pronounced. Sound is incredibly important for communication, and not just through speech. The vibrations that sounds produce have the ability to harmonize dissonant frequencies within and around us.

When this chakra is balanced, we feel resonant with the world around us, empowered to speak our truth, a channel for Divine to work through us. Fifth chakra energy reminds us that when we do what's in highest and best for us, it's also in highest and best for all beings.

Experiences that can cause this chakra to be closed off or in need of attention and strengthening:

- Being silenced by your peers, partner, or caregiver

- Feeling like you were never given the chance to be heard

- Feeling like your opinions don't matter

- Fearing what others would think about you if you spoke what was on your mind or in your heart

The throat chakra gets "inflamed" when unexpressed energy is held back and in. Think about any time you had a sore throat, laryngitis, or any other issue where it hurt to talk or you lost your voice. When the throat is swollen, it's not only hard to speak, but often actually hurts, too.

While one of shungite's healing properties is promoting stronger immunity, it also acts as an energetic anti-inflammatory. Shungite helps absorb any energetic irritation or negativity caused by "holding our tongue" or not speaking our mind, emboldening us with a desire for our voice to be heard, allowing the vibration of our voice to sound full and confident.

Because of its link to communication, the throat chakra awards us the ability to become aware of things on a vibrational level. If there is a blockage in this area, working with shungite can help us better determine when something is in or out of sync in our surroundings, which enables us to make more resonant, aligned choices for ourselves.

USING SHUNGITE TO SUPPORT YOUR THROAT CHAKRA

If you're looking for help to heal and clear your fifth chakra, wearing a shungite necklace is a great way to keep the powerful mineral on and around your throat. You may forget that you're even wearing it from time to time, so to be intentional about what you are doing, create a ceremony out of putting it on by stating your intention for healing this area each time you secure it around your neck.

Examples of affirmations or intentions for the throat chakra:

- I communicate my needs to others

- I contribute great ideas and solutions at home and at work

- I have strong boundaries that keep me healthy and safe

- I speak clearly and with intention

- Saying no to someone else is saying yes to myself

 ## SING YOUR THROAT CHAKRA OUT

One of my favorite ways to clear the fifth chakra is to sing. Singing helps you get used to hearing your own voice, which will make you feel more confident to speak up and let your voice be heard when it's needed. Create a playlist with all your favorite songs to play while you're in the shower, cleaning your home, getting ready for work, or even cooking. Grab your harmonizers to sing into like they're your microphones and let yourself have fun rocking out to your favorite jams.

 ## (BOOSTED) SPIRAL GRID

Imbalances found in the sacral and throat chakras are often linked, so the grid for the throat chakra is similar, but with a twist.

1. Place a large piece of shungite (a pyramid, sphere, or tower are best, but any piece will work) in the middle.

2. Using any other crystals you have, draw five or more (whatever space and the number of crystals you have

allow) lines from the center that curve, creating a flower-like shape.

3. Write your intention on a piece of paper, fold it up, and place it under the center stone.

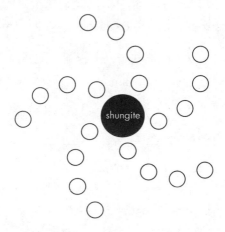

SIXTH CHAKRA • THIRD EYE CHAKRA • AJNA

Location: the third eye, the space between the eyebrows

Association: clarity, truth, clear vision, clear knowing (knowing something without any history or prior relationship to the thing); it's referred to as "the third eye" because it enables us to know, see, and understand things beyond the logical, rational mind; the sixth sense

Governs: the pineal gland

Because it's located in the brain, the sixth chakra is more cerebral than the lower chakras. Often referred to as "the seat of the soul," the pineal gland responds to variations in light by secreting hormones through the autonomic nervous system, the regulator of involuntary functions such as heart rate, blood pressure, and digestion. It's also the manager of your circadian rhythms: if the pineal gland senses it's dark, melatonin is produced, signaling to the body that it's time to sleep; it helps keep you awake and alert if it senses light.

The openness and development of the sixth chakra allow us to remove our personal blinders that cloud our judgments and perceptions of the world in order for us to not only see the bigger picture but also become a part of it, penetrating the illusions we've created for ourselves. It's here that we become conscious, which helps us understand that we can deliberately choose to break away from any negative habits, attitudes, or thoughts that we've been living by and replace them with new, supportive ones. This is why working with affirmations is so powerful: you may not believe them as you say them at first, but over time, if used regularly and repeatedly, the words you choose to hear, the words you *want to believe,* help to shift not just your perspective but your energy as well.

The sixth chakra awakens us to the universal truth that we are all connected, that, together, we are part of something bigger. Governing our power to choose, when this energy center is open and in alignment, we're able to make informed decisions for ourselves, and we realize that whatever is in highest and best for us is also in highest and best for all beings and the world.

Because of the location of this chakra, it's often called "the third eye." While our eyes help us to understand where we are physically in relation to our surroundings in order to move and interact with the world around us, the sixth chakra helps us to contextualize all that our eyes cannot; it's our window into a higher wisdom, the seat of our intuition, our sixth sense.

Experiences that can cause this chakra to be closed off or in need of attention and strengthening:

- Being made fun of for "knowing" something that hasn't happened yet

- Not being encouraged to trust or follow your intuitive hits, feelings, or visions

- Experiencing a lack of support or encouragement in trusting your extrasensory perception

- Fearing others will think you're weird or strange because you felt or saw something they didn't

- Lacking boundaries with use of electronics

- Looking at your cell phone, watching TV, playing video games, or using anything with a light-up screen right before bedtime

- Anxiety

Intuition is defined as the ability to understand something immediately, without the need for conscious reasoning; it's your higher Self trying to connect with your earthly self to steer you toward your purpose. It doesn't speak to you like your thoughts do. Where your thoughts are loud, intuition is more a whisper, a knowing, a feeling. And it's easy to miss if you've been told to ignore it, because the people you trusted to look out for you and take care of you told you it wasn't there. Once you stop looking for it, you miss it altogether.

Everyone has their own language(s) with their intuition; your intuition won't speak to you or grab your attention the same way every time it's trying to get you to listen, which is why you have to develop a relationship with it to understand when it is trying to come through.

Tuning in to our intuition feels most accessible when we're calm, getting enough sleep, and our digestion is functioning properly. This can feel challenging or downright impossible when we're feeling anxious. Anxiety, as we'll discuss in the next chapter, affects all of these functions. It feels like internal chaos, which keeps us from feeling anything but calm. There's no way we can tune in or be able to see the bigger picture and our place in it if we can't ground anxious energy.

Shungite's ability to calm anxiety, depression, and stress helps to clear the mind of any extra outside noise that keeps us from listening inward. Plus, its ability to neutralize EMFs, which contribute to our feelings of anxiety, helps us to feel more grounded and discover a sense of peace. It's from a quieter, more peaceful place that we are better able to tune in to our intuition, enabling us to live a more embodied life that allows us to trust the messages that come through.

USING SHUNGITE TO SUPPORT YOUR THIRD EYE CHAKRA

Having shungite in your home will naturally aid in strengthening your sixth chakra. But if you are looking for a more active way to work with it to give your intuition a boost and help bring on a sweet sense of calm, take a tumbled piece of shungite in either hand and gently trace your eyebrows from the bridge of your nose and massage toward your temples. Repeat this motion five to seven times—or more if you're feeling it—and then sit in silence and stillness for a few moments afterward to notice any shifts in your mindset or how you are feeling.

Examples of affirmations or intentions for the third eye chakra:

- I see my past experiences as necessary life lessons I had to learn from

- I forgive my past in order to see the role I play in the bigger picture

- I trust my intuition

- I am open to the wisdom that lies within me

- My thoughts create my reality

 FIREWORK GRID

Similar to the star grid we made for the power chakra, we'll start with a centerpiece and, depending on how many crystals you have, radiate multiple lines from the center. However, instead of closing up the circle like we did for the power chakra, keep the lines open. Intuitive energy cannot be contained, so our grid reflects this to help us stay open to receiving.

1. Place a large piece of shungite (a pyramid, sphere, or tower are best, but any piece will work) in the middle.

2. Create lines with smaller crystals that grow away from the centerpiece.

3. Place larger crystals at the end of each line.

4. Write your intention on a piece of paper and place it underneath the centerpiece.

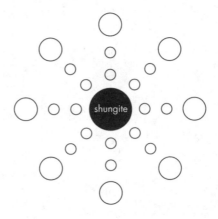

SEVENTH CHAKRA • CROWN CHAKRA • SAHASRARA

Location: hovers over the crown of the head

Association: centeredness, awareness, thought, intelligence, the ability to recognize patterns in our lives, inspiration; connection to the whole self, source energy, nature, and all that is around us

Governs: the pituitary gland; regulates growth hormone; activates the thyroid; activates adrenals, follicle-stimulating hormone, sex hormones, prolactin, endorphins, enkephalins, beta-melanocyte-stimulating hormone, vasopressin, oxytocin

The sixth chakra allows us to see the bigger picture, but it's the seventh chakra that helps us integrate our life experiences to give a sense of meaning to our lives.

When it feels like we have purpose, that our lives have meaning, we feel a sense of belonging, a strong connection not just to ourselves but to everything around us. It's in our nature to feel a connection to ourselves and what's around us because all the elements that exist around us—earth, air, fire, and water—also exist within us. Our biofield mimics the earth's. If we can't find meaning in what we do or are unable to connect to others in a deep, meaningful way, it can feel like something is lacking in our lives, which could propel us into an endless search for meaning and connection.

The crown is symbolic of higher wisdom. Crowns remind us of royalty or persons in positions of power. Knowledge equals power. Hovering over the body, this chakra acts like an antenna picking up signals from the world around us. It's more than just conscious, intellectual knowledge. What we've learned intellectually is mixed with, or enhanced by, the somatic wisdom of the body as well as an awareness of Divine: how things feel, sensations.

How information makes its way to us is similar to crystal formation. In Chapter One we learned that magma has no order, that within magma there is a plethora of different mineral-forming substances that come together to create all the different minerals and crystals that exist on Earth. Similarly, before outside information gets to us, it is orderless. Once we pick up on it, it comes into our consciousness, where it falls into a pattern within our energy, like a crystal lattice. Yet another instance of human life imitating nature.

One of the most powerful lessons of the seventh chakra is learning that things happen *for* us, not *to* us. We can choose to find the meaning in something, noticing the habits we've fallen into and seeing repeating patterns in our thoughts, reactions, and relationships; we can notice how these are reflections of our personal conditioning, manifestations of how our energy has been steering us because of the experiences we've lived through. Or we can choose to believe we are unlucky, that bad things happen for no reason, ignoring the symbolism and lessons each experience—good and bad—affords us.

Our minds are wildly powerful and prove our self-fulfilling prophecies over and over again. We can choose to see things negatively if we feel bad or depressed, or we can decide to look for the silver lining.

Experiences that can cause this chakra to be closed off or in need of attention and strengthening:

- Depression
- Feelings of being alone, unsupported, ostracized, or unaccepted
- Following a teacher whose message is not in alignment with you or the universe
- Being a part of a group or job whose energy, message, or purpose is not in line with yours or the universe

There is no way to access our intuition or discover clarity if the mind is in overdrive, thinking too many things at once. It's unable to make sense of the information it's taking in, which can feel like a jumble of thoughts moving so fast that it's hard to know what is right for us or which thoughts to hold on to if we don't already have a strong sense of Self.

Since shungite helps promote the exchange of information between neurotransmitters, it helps us make sense of the messages and information that come to and through us. Its grounding abilities are helpful in drawing energy and information in and down into the body for it to be assimilated and processed, helping to enhance our feelings of interconnectedness with the world around us.

USING SHUNGITE TO SUPPORT YOUR CROWN CHAKRA

To help open the crown chakra, we'll give the kundalini ego eradicator exercise an update by using harmonizers to help you feel more grounded through this active breathing practice. Kundalini is a style of yoga that focuses heavily on meditation and breathing exercises coupled with specific movements and postures to transform energy and expand consciousness. We use the ego eradicator to help clear the mind and bring us into a heightened state of awareness.

1. Come to a comfortable seat, rooting your tailbone down toward the earth, the crown of your head extending upward toward the sky.

2. Holding harmonizers in your hands, create a *V* shape with your arms as you reach them toward the sky.

3. With the eyes closed, breathe short, sharp breaths out the nose. Focus on the out breath; the inhale will naturally come on its own. Try to contain any movements to the pumping of the belly as you breathe.

4. Continue to breathe like this with the arms extended for 3 minutes then release your arms down, resting your hands on your lap.

5. Notice any shifts of clarity in the mind or openness around the top of the head.

Examples of affirmations or intentions for the crown chakra:

- Divine exists within me
- I am connected to all things
- I am in co-creation with Divine
- I trust that I am exactly where I need to be
- Magic is possible

 CONNECT-TO-THE-COSMOS GRID

Here is a grid that focuses on the crown chakra. You may want to grab all of your crystals for this one.

1. Place the largest piece of shungite you have (a pyramid or tower is best, but any piece will work) closest to you on your table or gridding space.

2. Then, with as many crystals as you like, start to place them above the first main piece you put down to make it look like crystal energy is pouring into the crown chakra.

3. Write your intention on a piece of paper and place it underneath your shungite, the first crystal you put down to create this grid.

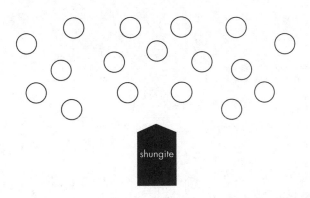

You can also draw the template for this grid shape and place it under the crystals of your grid. Think of it as a blueprint or map. This will help bring more of your energy and intention into the grid and empower it with the thought you put into your design that was born out of the intention you had in mind. Let it sit for at least one to two days, or however long you'd like.

PUTTING IT ALL TOGETHER

Our life experiences determine not just how we interact with the world, but the energy of each chakra. As we've explored each energy center, we have seen just how much our external world affects our internal processes. Transformation can't happen unless we have an understanding of the factors in our lives that have made a tremendous impact on us and a tenacious desire to change—it's an honest awareness of our strengths and weaknesses.

The inner structures of metamorphic minerals like shungite become stronger because the immense heat and pressure thrust upon them force the weaker substances out. Similarly, when we embark on our own transformation, the parts of ourselves that can no longer stand the heat—old habits, emotional patterns, inherited or learned conditioning—burn away as we awaken to how they have held us back from living out our dreams and fully embodying the person we were meant to be.

We have so much to learn from our pain, yet we treat it like it's an intruder, something that shouldn't be there. Our personal struggles are necessary parts of our journey, key parts to our own personal metamorphosis. When we understand that the old way isn't working, we begin to question everything and initiate an intense self-reflection that takes a metaphoric magnifying glass to our core values. What we realize no longer works or we no longer find acceptable gives way to new values that feel more aligned with our soul. Shift or get off the pot.

Crystals and chakras are inherently linked because both function energetically. In fact, the chakras act as portals for a crystal's energy to enter the body and circulate through your aura and energetic pathways, helping to bring your entire being into balance.

If you're experiencing a mental or emotional block, feeling stuck in certain areas of your life, or are in the throes of a particularly difficult time or phase, placing crystals directly on and/or around the energy centers can help restore balance energetically, which can also help you find balance in the world around you. When you experience balance inside yourself, everything around you will seem to fall into place.

Was there a particular chakra description that spoke to you when reading through this chapter? If so, lay a piece of shungite on top of the energy center for as long as feels right to you. I suggest a minimum of 5 minutes, but you can decide the length if you want to go longer.

Feel free to work on more than one chakra at a time in this way. If you think more than one needs your attention and have multiple pieces of shungite or other crystals on hand, you can place as many on yourself as you like.

PRACTICES TO CLEAR AND CONNECT ALL YOUR CHAKRAS

If you're looking to maximize your abilities and affect all your chakras at once, try your hand at either of these exercises to help clear all the chakras at once.

 ## MERKABAH GRID

If you think of the lower three chakras as a triangle pointed upward and the upper three chakras as a triangle pointed downward, they unite in the middle, where the fourth chakra sits, creating a *merkabah*. The *merkabah* is a three-dimensional Star of David. A Hebrew word, it phonetically translates from ancient Egyptian as "light, body, spirit"—the merging of the three. To help bring balance and harmony to all your chakras, we'll use this shape for a more elaborate grid.

1. Draw one triangle pointing up and one triangle pointing down to create the *merkabah* shape on a piece of paper or cloth.

2. Place a piece of shungite in the middle of the overlapping triangles to represent the heart chakra for your centerpiece.

3. Place six pieces of shungite or other larger crystals that you have on the corners of the triangles.

4. Write your intention on a piece of paper and place it under the central shungite.

5. If you have a crystal point or wand, tap the top of the crystal representing the heart chakra and then tap one of the corner crystals to connect their energy.

6. Repeat, tapping the heart chakra crystal before tapping each of the other crystals to connect them all.

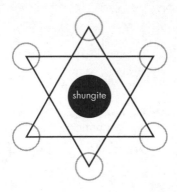

 ## GROUNDING CORD MEDITATION FOR ALL CHAKRAS

Similar to the recommended meditation for the root chakra, this exercise includes breathing earth energy into all the chakras to help clear, balance, and support them.

1. Come to a comfortable seat, rooting your tailbone down toward the earth, the crown of your head extending upward toward the sky.

2. Close your eyes and let your breath come naturally, noticing your breathing for a few moments.

3. Start to bring your awareness to your tailbone, the base of your spine.

4. Imagine a cord growing out of your tailbone, lengthening and lowering down into the earth. Watch as it continues to move downward, further and further down toward the center of the earth.

5. On an inhale, envision drawing energy up the cord to your first chakra, located at the base of the spine.

6. Exhale the energy back down the cord to the earth.

7. Inhale energy back up the cord to your second chakra, located in the lower belly, a few inches below the navel; exhale the energy back down to the earth.

8. Inhale energy back up the cord to your third chakra, located at the solar plexus, above the belly button, near the lower ribs; exhale the energy back down to the earth.

9. Inhale energy back up the cord to your fourth chakra, located at the heart center; exhale the energy back down to the earth.

10. Inhale energy back up the cord to your fifth chakra, located at the base of the throat; exhale the energy back down to the earth.

11. Inhale energy back up the cord to your sixth chakra, located at the space between the eyebrows; exhale the energy back down to the earth.

12. Inhale energy back up the cord to your seventh chakra, located at the crown of the head; exhale the energy back down to the earth.

13. Repeat the last step, drawing energy up through the body, passing through all the chakras back up to the crown of the head on the inhale, sending energy back to the earth on the exhale two more times.

14. Let your breath come back to its regular pace, letting the cord go. Notice how you feel after using the breath to help clear and open each chakra.

Shungite is incredibly effective in helping us access and strengthen the first three chakras, which also tend to be the hardest chakras to heal because of how deeply embedded their programming is and how deeply it affects us. Shungite's powerful stabilizing force helps to anchor us into the work with the first three chakras because of its receptive yin qualities.

Having shungite around our homes can help us to better focus our attention inward, not only to see which chakras need tending to, but also to help us understand what's ours in the energy that we sense all around us, what's electric, and what we might be picking up from others. It can help detoxify our thoughts as we begin to clean up shop, aiding our process to radically shift our perspective on our own stories, the lives of the other characters in our stories, and everything that happens around us. Being able to see and feel more clearly, we begin to rewire our internal systems to choose differently for ourselves for our highest good in order to live a more fulfilled, purposeful life.

CHAPTER 7

Anxiety

After diving into the subtle energy bodies of our aura and the chakras, it's clear that human beings have a special ability to sense things when in conversation, in close proximity to another human, or even without the need for words. Whether we realize we're doing it or not, we pick up cues from witnessing the tension in a person's face, their eye movements, or the pitch and fluctuations of their voice. These act as clues for us to determine how the other person is feeling. The autonomic nervous system interprets them, alerting us to whether it's safe to stay or if we're in danger and need to get out of there as soon as possible.

Humans regularly sense the energy of our external world. We want to be accepted; we seek approval; we want to feel as if we are important. From the day we are born we start learning what garners us praise and what elicits punishment. This affects our strengths as well as our potential hang-ups. Whatever we learned or inherited from our caregivers, traumatic experiences, or interactions from our formative years affect the vibrations of the chakras.

Intuition is something that we all have access to, yet it has become increasingly challenging for many to connect with. Have you ever heard someone say they had a "gut feeling" about something? Intuition doesn't just speak to us through our minds, but as feelings to help us differentiate between our thoughts and what's real. For those of us who suffer anxiety, we feel things profoundly, but since we pick up on so much it's hard to tell whether what we feel is our own energy or someone else's. It's hard to trust our gut if we don't trust what we feel. Anxiety lives in the belly; it's often what blocks us from accessing our intuition.

Twenty years into the twenty-first century, anxiety is so well-known, it's basically a celebrity. Something that's been on everyone's minds, lips, and TV show story lines, it's come a long way since the Betty Draper days of the early '60s, when it was something only talked about in secret. This disease mysteriously appeared right around the time the world began to be electrified, wrapped by millions of miles of telegraph wires, like a Christmas tree entangled in twinkle lights. Is it merely coincidence that this phenomenon erupted in our culture around the same time humans first came in constant contact with electricity?

First labeled neurasthenia, its symptoms correlated with the descriptions of those who say they are environmentally and electronically sensitive today: fatigue, confusion, insomnia, muscle and joint pain, and increased difficulties in everyday functions. These symptoms began to pop up among many different types of people, no matter their social status, for no discernable reason. In 1895, Austrian neurologist and founder of psychoanalysis Sigmund Freud renamed the malady anxiety neurosis.

Today, anxiety affects nearly 20 percent of the world population and is ranked as the most common mental illness in the United States, affecting more than forty million people.[14] It's commonly experienced as excessive worry or dread, irrational fears, repetitive thoughts, apprehension, neurosis, and social phobias. It's something you can't put your finger on. It's constantly shifting and changing, but it always leaves you in a constant state of want, working yourself up into a vicious frenzy of thinking about all possible scenarios, planning for specific outcomes for future threatening events that 9.8 times out of ten don't come to pass. It's an inability to tolerate or accept uncertainty. What will happen? Who am I going to talk to? What will I say that will wow and amaze others so that I am accepted?

Being in a state of anxiety is the brain's defense mechanism in response to a predator or predatory experience, a response to a possible threat that may or may not happen. It's thinking about the future, how to get out of a tight situation.

Let's be clear that experiencing anxiety is a totally normal, natural function of life. We are meant to feel it from time to time. It's when it occurs frequently, with uncontrollable excessive intensity, and for long, sometimes unending lengths of time—to the extent it disrupts daily life—that there is cause for concern.

---

14   Jamie Ducharme, "A Lot of Americans Are More Anxious than They Were Last Year, a New Poll Says," *Time*, May 8, 2018, https://time.com/5269371/americans-anxiety-poll.

Pay attention to these adjectives used to describe anxiety: frenzied, shifting, changing, planning, unsettled, nervous, fidgety. Anxious energy *moves*. That is how it lives and thrives within the human body. It darts around inside, moving through different organs, disrupting their functions, and quite literally creating physical dis-ease.

Traditional Chinese medicine allocates different emotions to different organs of the body; the liver is tied to anger, the kidneys fear, the spleen excessive worry, the lungs grief and anxiety. We learned in Chapter Five how the breath affects the strength of our aura; it also plays a pivotal role in how we experience anxiety. Funny how breathing—a function we don't even have to think about that literally gives us life—is connected to our health in so many invisible ways. So maybe we should consider it more? Let's take a closer look.

NOTICE YOUR BREATH

Take a moment to notice your breath right now.

Where do you feel your breath moving? What parts of your body move because of your breath? Notice the lengths of your breath. How long are your inhales? How long are your exhales?

Most people tend to only notice the breath moving the chest around the heart space. Unless we pause to think about it, we unconsciously take short, shallow breaths. Breathing terse, restricted breaths actually adds to that general feeling of uneasiness, creating more anxiety. I'll explain.

The human body was designed with the capacity to breathe in diverse ways to help us regulate our nervous system. The sympathetic nervous system (SNS) is the accelerator, the strength behind our fight-or-flight response. Roman physician Galen named it as such some two thousand years ago after discovering evidence that linked the SNS with our emotions. When the SNS is turned on, it pulls resources from all over the body, jump-starting the adrenal glands to shoot adrenaline into the bloodstream, pumping that blood to the muscles for quick action, speeding up the heart, and increasing blood pressure to get you out of a hairy situation fast.

The parasympathetic nervous system (PNS), on the other hand, slows things down, restores balance, and brings the body back to homeostasis. It governs our digestive functions, helps our wounds heal, relaxes our muscles, and slows our breath and heart rate. For those of us who exist in a constant state of anxiety, the PNS is unable to turn on and stay on long enough—if at all—to slow us down, calm us down, and pull us out of our heightened state. Shungite's calming effects allow us to deepen our breath, activating the PNS to help us self-soothe the SNS to balance and stabilize our energy systems.

 ## EXPERIMENT WITH YOUR BREATH

Close your eyes and take a few short, quick breaths in and out the nose. You'll notice that your heart rate begins to increase. Now, keeping the eyes closed, take a few elongated breaths. Breathe in for a count of four and breathe out for a count of four, focusing on lengthening the exhale as you breathe out the mouth. You'll notice the heart rate start to slow, and you'll feel a more overall sense of calm as you continue to breathe in and out in counts of four. If you have a piece or two of shungite, try this breathing exercise a second time while holding your crystals and notice the difference between how you felt without the shungite and how you feel holding it.

◇◇◇

The length of our breaths directly affects our anxious or composed states. If you regularly take short, quick breaths, this shortness of breath sends a message to the brain and all other energy systems of the body that something isn't right, which alerts the nervous system that it's go time, that we're in danger and need to get out of there quick, so all our energy is sent to our mind and our limbs to power us through whatever is standing in the way of our safety. Think back to the previous chapters where we discussed the importance of the breath to our aura and power chakra. Our breath is linked to the strength of both. Put simply, modern-day anxiety quite literally robs us of our power.

A NATURAL SURVIVAL TOOL

Biologically, anxiety is meant to put you in a heightened state of awareness to keep you on your toes should you encounter a potential threat. It's that sixth-sense extrasensory perception that lets you know when something is off, that something's wrong, that danger is near. Think about the reaction of deer in the woods or squirrels in your yard when they sense your presence. Think of your dog or cat freezing up when the doorbell rings or someone they've never met comes into your home. They freeze up to allow all their senses to dial up to their maximum potential to judge whether or not what they heard or sensed is a threat.

Anxiety's fight-or-flight function is the same for humans, a survival tool to help us sense when danger is afoot.

Freezing is another important survival mechanism. In fact, this is usually our first response when we detect a possible threat. Many predators use movement to track their prey, and so we instinctively freeze when we sense something is off. Think of the T. Rex scene in *Jurassic Park*: paleontologist Alan Grant sits in the second Jeep urging the scared kids in the first Jeep to be still so that the dinosaur will pass by without detecting them. In real life, we stop whatever we are doing in order for our senses to take in information to decide whether we can make a run for it or if we have to fight. This is literally where we get the phrase "deer in the headlights" from: it's describing someone who freezes in a heightened state of awareness in much the same way a deer freezes in place when crossing a street at night and all of a sudden a car is upon them.

We've come a long way since our days of fastening sharp stones to pieces of wood to make tools and weapons. We may no longer be running from saber-toothed tigers, but we still experience threats. Today they come in the form of emails from a boss or coworker unhappy with our work performance; fear of rejection by a partner, potential partner, friend, or potential employer; the ding of our phone with a text message, email, or social media notification possibly alerting us to either approval or dismissal from the people we know or, worse, complete strangers on the internet. And just like if we were in the woods and realized a bear was nearby, we freeze when we receive these "threats," eyes wide, our breath short and shallow. How do we respond? We avoid, ignore, or ghost (our modern-day version of flight), or we shoot off a text or email in our defense, aka fight.

When catapulted into a fight, flight, or freeze response, systems of the body that aren't an immediate priority, such as digestion, elimination, growth, repair/sleep, and reproduction, are shut down to conserve and redistribute energy to where it can best be used to protect itself.

Anyone who experiences anxiety often or has been diagnosed with an anxiety disorder likely has experienced constipation, irritable bowel syndrome (IBS), insomnia, or reproductive issues. You'll notice that these are all related to the systems that get turned off when the body is in a heightened state preparing to run or fight. Today roughly 63 million American adults suffer from chronic constipation; 11 percent of the world population suffers from IBS;[15] one in three Americans don't get proper sleep, and one out of four Americans develop insomnia each year;[16] and infertility issues exist in at least 6 million women in the US[17] and 30

15   National Institute of Diabetes and Digestive and Kidney Diseases, "Digestive Diseases Statistics for the United States," November 1, 2014, https://www.niddk .nih.gov/health-information/health-statistics/digestive-diseases.
16   University of Pennsylvania School of Medicine, "One in Four Americans Develop Insomnia Each Year: 75 Percent of Those with Insomnia Recover," *ScienceDaily*, June 8, 2018, https://www.sciencedaily.com/releases/2018/06/180605154114.htm.
17   Office on Women's Health, "Infertility," updated April 1, 2019, https://www.womenshealth.gov/a-z-topics/infertility.

million men worldwide.[18] Chances are, if you don't suffer from one of these ailments, you know someone who does.

THE LINK BETWEEN ANXIETY AND AIR

Ayurveda is one of the oldest known holistic healing systems. Sanskrit for "the science of life," it originated in India over three thousand years ago and looks to digestion to determine our overall health. It acknowledges the active elemental forces of nature—air, fire, water—are also the elemental forces of the body: *vata*, *pitta*, *kapha*, respectively. Known as the doshas, meaning "fault" or "blemish," factors that, if disturbed, can bring about disease and decay, each exhibits different physical traits and qualities and is related to specific areas and functions of the body. A balance is needed between the three, but depending on a person's constitution or current state of health, there can be an imbalance with one, two, or even all three doshas.

Anxiety is intrinsically linked to *vata*, the ruler of all the doshas. Since it's governed by air, *vata* is the principle of mobility for all the body's processes and functions. *Vata* also regulates respiration, circulation, metabolism, digestion, elimination, thought, and movement. It's responsible for sensory, emotional, and mental harmony. *Vata* helps us process information and inspires creativity. It also enables messages to be sent via nerve synapses.

---

18   Ashok Agarwal et al., "A Unique View on Male Infertility around the Globe," *Reproductive Biology and Endocrinology*, April 26, 2015, https://doi.org/10.1186/s12958-015-0032-1.

We mentioned earlier that anxiety likes to move; *vata* moves things. When there's too much *vata*, it's hard to sit still, circulation is poor, we walk quicker, we feel spacey, we forget things, we find it hard to commit to things, and we experience digestion issues, tending toward constipation.

Pitta, governed by fire, is the transforming element. It needs *vata* to get things moving and help stoke the digestive fires. It's the force that regulates body temperature, absorption, thirst, understanding, and metabolism; it's the force that digests our food. Its highly fiery nature can arouse anger, hatred, and jealousy when "heated." Those with a predominant *pitta* constitution can be seen as competitive, aggressive, and judgmental. In balance, *pitta* promotes understanding, intelligence, and reasoning; out of balance, it produces tension and stress.

Kapha is governed by water, the stabilizer, the binder; its function is to lubricate in order to make things stick together. Think mucus and plasma. It hydrates and nourishes all tissues in the body. It needs *vata* to be stimulated to move; *pitta* is necessary for warmth. If water is cold and/or stagnant, it is unable to provide life. *Kapha*'s capacity to "hold" makes it a force that provides strength and stability. When in balance, *kapha* is expressed as love, calmness, forgiveness, and connection. Out of balance *kapha* leads to attachment, greed, and envy.

Vata is the motivating force for *pitta* and *kapha*. It fans the flames of fire for *pitta*, fueling its drive to keep going; it inspires *kapha* to move to avoid stagnation. Without *vata*, their functions would come to a screeching halt, and they would be unable to successfully carry out their duties.

FIVE FORMS OF *VATA*

Since *vata* governs air in the body, it's important to know that within the body there are five different types of *vayus*, or winds, in which air moves.

1. *Prana* rules the chest and head. It is the air we breathe, the primary life force in the body. It maintains the heart, the lungs, and the act of swallowing. Its direction of flow is inward. Lack of concentration and difficulty accessing intuition are common side effects of *prana* imbalances. Meditating with shungite harmonizers in your hands for 5–10 minutes a day can help strengthen *prana* and enhance intuition.

2. *Udana* rules the throat, responsible not only for our exhalation and speech (the air that leaves our mouths) but also for the thyroid, the master of metabolism, which controls the body's cells to convert food into energy to fuel all the body's processes. It blows upward from within us. Breathing complications, nausea, and fear of expressing oneself are signs that *udana vayu* is compromised. If *udana vayu* is weak, you can lie down with a sphere of shungite resting on your throat chakra or refer back to the previous chapter for more fifth chakra exercises to help clear this area.

3. *Vyana* governs the circulatory system, the movement of joints and muscles, the flow of thoughts and feelings. Originating in the heart, it is an expansive wind, blowing in all directions. If the hands or feet are too cold, it's a sign

that circulation is poor and *vyana vayu* is not strong enough. You can take a tumbled piece of shungite and, starting at the heart, radiate outward in all directions as you gently make contact with your skin, massaging yourself to help increase circulation: down the arms, down the torso and legs, up toward the throat and the crown of the head.

4. *Samana* balances. Centered in the small intestine, it's the force that controls digestion. It swirls and churns in the belly in a clockwise motion. Too much of this *vata* can put out the *pitta* fire that is necessary for digestion. To strengthen, take a tumbled piece of shungite directly to your belly and move in the same direction *samana vayu* moves in: clockwise. Do this for 1 minute, or longer if time allows.

5. *Apana* lives in the colon, *vata's* primary location, and governs all processes of elimination. It moves out and down. For those who err on the side of constipation, it's a sign *apana vayu* is too weak (too much *vata*) to move waste from the body. To strengthen, trace imaginary lines from your navel down all sides of your legs toward your feet, culminating at your heels or toes. If you tend toward diarrhea, *apana vayu* is too strong (too much *pitta*). To balance, take a tumbled piece of shungite and trace an imaginary line from your toes and heel to your navel in an upward motion; do this from multiple angles of your foot so that you trace up the front, sides, and back of your legs.

Excess *vata* causes digestive issues as well as mental and nervous disorders that often manifest as anxiety. With five different winds blowing within the body, it's no wonder that, if there is an imbalance, it can feel like we're being pulled in many different directions at once, like it's hard to sit still or think straight, or like there is a noticeable uneasiness in the belly. Understanding how air moves in the body, it's clear that anxiety can physically affect us in subtle, energetic ways.

FROM THE OUTSIDE IN

From an energetic perspective, if the energy within ourselves is already excited, the energy around us will have an impact. And vice versa: if there is excitable energy around us, it will excite the energy within us.

With advances in technology, the pace of everything we do has quickened. The high speed of the internet and broad-band cellular network technology necessary to power our computers, smartphones, and Wi-Fi–connected toys affects the speed at which energy moves within us, adding to anxiety levels and making us feel even more frazzled. The high speed of our electronics isn't only affecting how quickly information gets to us; it also creates the expectation of a faster output from us and adds an invisible pressure to constantly be *doing*.

We see this fast pace especially in cities, which already have an excitable energy about them. With more buildings, more cars, more jobs, more people, more electricity being used (not only to power people's homes and jobs but also to operate infrastructure like traffic signals, street lights, and subway systems), life literally feels as if it's moving ten times faster in cities than in the suburbs and more rural parts of the world. And with larger populations and so much going on in them, they are quite literally moving at a faster pace than areas less densely populated.

Washington, DC, the capital of the US, feels infused with an energetic urgency. People walk so fast you wouldn't be alone in thinking that some folks were about to break into a run. Is it any wonder that, with so many lawyers, politicians, and nonprofits, a majority of those who live and work here are literally trying to change the world?

New York City, on the other hand, has a more creative energy. And rightfully so: it's been the go-to destination for journalists, dancers, musicians, and performers for decades as the city that attracts millions with its promise of making dreams come true. Remember that imaginative, creative energy is the stuff of *vata* and the sixth and seventh chakras. With 1.6 million people living on an island that's only 22.7 square miles, the "City That Never Sleeps" (insomnia being a side effect of too much *vata* and anxious energy) got its nickname from the millions of visionaries who've descended on the concrete jungle to push themselves tooth and nail to manifest their goals into reality.

With so much active energy surrounding city dwellers, not to mention so much more noise and light pollution (artificial light), it's no wonder those who live in more densely populated areas are particularly sensitive to their surroundings. A 2009 Dutch study found that those living in a city were 21 percent more likely to develop an anxiety disorder.[19] Which

---

19   J. Peen et al., "The Current Status of Urban-Rural Differences in Psychiatric Disorders," *Acta Psychiatrica Scandinavica* 121, no. 2 (2009): 84–93, https://pubmed.ncbi.nlm.nih.gov/19624573.

gives any city dweller more of an excuse to keep a pyramid of shungite under the bed and a tumbled piece in their pocket at all times.

SO HOW DO WE TREAT ANXIETY?

If anxious energy moves, the antidote is to slow it down. The word *grounding* gets thrown around a lot in yoga and healing communities. For those of us who need it most, its meaning might not seem obvious. When we talk about "grounding our energy," what we're really saying is that we're trying to calm and stabilize it. Because the energy of anxiety is erratic, it's hard to sit still, which then makes it challenging to focus.

If you think of the word *ground* and what it actually is and does, you realize that the soil nurtures and nourishes the plants that grow out of it with nutrients and minerals. It's solid and reliable in that it is always there. It provides a foundation for the homes we live in. It supports us in every step that we take. Anxious energy is balanced by inviting in its opposite energy.

Since crystals come from the earth, they are naturally grounding, one reason why shungite is a helpful tool in calming anxious energy. Shungite is classified as a yin mineral, and whenever you hold, wear, or stand or sit next to a piece of it, you can't help but notice a strong sense of calm wash over you. This is the antidote to anxious energy: peace, calmness, stillness, and stability, all of which feel more within our reach if we have shungite around to help us tap into these receptive qualities.

Easy ways to ground your energy:

- Commit to a daily meditation practice with a shungite sphere or harmonizer in either hand

- Meditate sitting in the grass or on the earth

- Orient yourself with your surroundings, checking in with all five of the senses: notice what is touching you (the fabric of your clothes, what you're standing or sitting on) and what you smell, hear, see, and taste

- Self-massage

- Stand with your bare feet in the grass or on the earth

- Visit a body of water—the ocean, a lake, a river—and sit on the earth while gazing out at the water

MEDITATION

Meditation is one of the most powerful tools to bring a sense of calm and curb anxiety. Whether you have a regular meditation practice or are just starting out, incorporating shungite into your sittings can dramatically enhance your experience.

Many people think that the point of meditation is to stop thinking. Unless you've been meditating for eighteen hours a day for the last thirty years, it's just not going to happen. Meditation offers us the opportunity to observe how our mind operates, to take note of thoughts as they pop up but not to get pulled in or attached to them. The more we sit with ourselves, the more we are able to understand our mind's habits and the better chance we have at not letting ourselves get lured into the various rabbit holes that take us out of the present moment. When we practice being present for a few minutes daily, it helps us to stay more in the moment when we're not meditating, bringing more ease into our day and quieting the storm of anxiety within us.

One of the easiest ways to actively work with shungite and intentionally incorporate its healing powers into your everyday life is to meditate with it. Whether you are new to meditating or already have a regular practice, integrating shungite into your contemplative practice is an effective way to find more peace and stillness in your practice.

Using spheres in both hands or a harmonizer in each hand (mixing the shapes makes the energy on either side uneven), sit down for your practice. If you choose to work with the harmonizers, hold the black shungite harmonizer in your left hand, as the left side is connected to yin, feminine, more receptive energy; hold the gray steatite harmonizer in your right hand, the side associated with yang, solar, more active energy. Together they work to help these energies that move within us to find balance and discover a sense of lightness and inner peace when working with them.

If you are new to meditation, set a timer for just 5 minutes and add 1 minute every week until you get to 10 minutes. Some days the time will fly by, others it will feel like ages. And that is why it's called practice: each time we sit is a new opportunity to observe our thoughts when it feels like we are doing it right as well as when we can't wait for it to be over. The goal of meditation isn't to stop our thoughts but to become observers of them when they arise. So sit and just let yourself notice what comes up, if you get pulled into a story the mind might be trying to distract you with, or if you're able to extricate yourself from the story or the rabbit holes the mind tries to lure you into.

PAIN RELIEF: SHUNGITE POWDER

Because of its anti-inflammatory effects, shungite can help reduce physical aches and joint pain. *Vata* rules the joints. When there is excess air in the body, it can get stuck in the joints because joints are the sites of movement; they are not fixed points. Every joint is surrounded by pockets of negative space so that bones can move with ease, but these are also sites that can become dry and cold to the point of cracking or even swelling.

You can purchase shungite powder or experiment with making your own.

Note: *I only recommend the DIY route with any particularly fragile pieces of elite shungite, pieces that seem brittle to the touch and easily crush under gentle pressure.*

1. Place a pinch or two of shungite powder in a small bowl or custard cup.

2. Whether you are DIYing it or buy it pre-crushed, add just enough filtered shungite water to make a paste with your powder. Think two parts powder, one part water.

3. Apply the paste to the affected areas of your body. To avoid getting black shungite powder stuck beneath your fingernails, apply it with a spoon, popsicle stick, or similar apparatus.

4. Using shungite this way, start slow, much like the way you built up a tolerance before introducing yourself to the powerful effects of your first larger piece. Leave the paste on for about 4–5 minutes. As you continue to work with the paste and your tolerance grows, let it stay on 1 minute more each time you apply.

Note: *This can get messy. It might be best to apply paste outside, over old newspapers, or in your bathtub or shower as the wet powder can leave residue on clothes, towels, blankets, etc. Stains will come out with common stain removers you may have in your home if you get it on rugs, towels, or your clothes.*

5. As you decide on where to wait it out before washing it off, keep in mind that the paste will flake off as it dries on you. If you don't use all of the paste up, no need to worry or throw it out. It will dry up, but adding a little more water to it will turn it right back into a paste.

FOOT MASSAGE

Reflexology is a type of massage system that associates different organs and systems of the body with different locations on the soles of your feet. Using small tumbled pieces of shungite to massage the soles of the feet has been found to help increase blood supply to different organs and tissues. Massaging your feet for 2–5 minutes daily can help manage blood pressure, relieve joint pain, and support bone health.

You can also use the stones to gently massage other areas of your body that feel achy, sore, or swollen.

SHUNGITE ROOM

If holding shungite brings on a sense of calm, imagine its effects on you when you're surrounded by it. Similar to salt rooms, a shungite room is completely covered in shungite: the floor, ceiling, and walls are all lined with tiles of the mineral.

What are the benefits of being completely surrounded by shungite? Spending time in a space where you're entirely enveloped by shungite will offer you the same benefits as having one or two crystals of it around—times a thousand. Just a few minutes spent sitting or lounging in a shungite room will help dramatically reduce anxiety and physical pain, stabilize blood pressure, noticeably decrease inflammation in any area of the body, restore vitality, and invigorate your aura, helping it expand substantially while also evaporating any lingering EMFs. You'll leave feeling clearheaded and renewed.

Shungite rooms may not become as ubiquitous as Starbucks, but they are growing in popularity as a destination for healing since the construction of one particular establishment in southern Russia. A shungite room was built in Beslan in 2006 for survivors of the 2004 Beslan school siege attack to visit as a way to help them heal psychologically. While medically approved and supported measures were taken by psychiatrists and psychologists to help the victims heal, it was clear that just a few sessions in the room made a noticeable difference when the disturbed children began drawing happy scenes with bright colors and learned to smile again.

If you're in a corner of the world that boasts a shungite room, check it out for a quick and easy way to take advantage of all the healing properties shungite boasts. During the visit, all you have to do is lounge away in the space.

Note: *Most establishments will likely have time limits to using a shungite room. This is both to make the space available to as many people as possible and for your own protection. If being in close proximity to a small piece for too long can bring on headaches and nausea for the energetically sensitive on first meetings, imagine how being completely surrounded by it might make you feel!*

While most shungite rooms are in Russia, there is one in the US and one in France:

US
The Angel Cooperative
51 Ethan Allen Highway
Ridgefield, CT 06877

France
La Roche Mère
7 Rue Gambey
75011 Paris

Conclusion: Looking to the Future with Shungite

It's unclear how the natives of Lake Onega first became aware of shungite's healing powers, and the details on how the Sumerians and ancient Egyptians knew of the restorative qualities of crystals are just as foggy. What is evident, however, is the reverence we human beings had for the elements around us, a respect for the energy and potential of things outside of ourselves. Before we looked to science for proof, we believed stones had certain catalytic properties because we saw that working with them enhanced our well-being.

As we continue to invent new technology to make our lives easier, the distance between us and our simpler, humble beginnings grows. Yet shungite's power remains the same, if not more compelling and more relevant than ever. Did nature know we'd desperately need this magic 2.5 billion years after creating it?

In an increasingly electrified world, shungite's ability to neutralize EMFs is the most powerful, natural antidote for our modern-day problems. When we can't focus because there are invisible streams of electricity buzzing around us, when we can't finish the task at hand because we're so worried about how it'll turn out or what other people think about it, when we can't sleep because we're so addicted to our phones that they are the last thing we look at before going to bed, stimulating the pineal gland to reduce the chances of getting a good night's sleep, shungite is the thing we can turn to to save us from ourselves.

As health insurance premiums continue to surge on an annual basis, the self-care industry—valued at a cool $10 billion,[20] perhaps in response to escalating health insurance costs—is thriving, attracting those empowered to take charge of their own health. Every day more people, from Gen Xers and millennials to baby boomers and those of the silent generation, commit to making healthier decisions for themselves in all areas of their lives. Self-care has become a collective awakening to the realization that for every action there is a reaction, that there are consequences that affect not just our physical health but our mindset as well.

Belief and expectation play a significant role when working with crystals. If this book is in your hands, my guess is that you already believe or want to believe they can enhance or help your life. Now more than ever natural alternatives to maintain and optimize health are becoming de rigueur as more and more people look to help themselves organically. It's my hope that some of the scientific data shared here has

---

20   Alice Hickson and Lilly Blumenthal, "The Self Care Obsession," *Tufts Observer*, March 25, 2019.

helped build your trust in the workings of our lives that seem to exist beyond the realm of plausibility.

To be clear, there is no one-size-fits-all approach to healing. The offerings and suggestions outlined in this book are just that: offerings and suggestions. Some may work as written about on the page, while others may empower you with curiosity, providing a jumping-off point from which you can follow through on a hunch or your intuition to try something different. But shungite's EMF-fighting, aura-enhancing, chakra-clearing, anxiety-relieving abilities cannot be overlooked; no matter its intended use, it's a powerful addition to everyone's self-care arsenal.

"Each time we choose to enhance our internal power, we limit the authority of the physical world over our lives, bodies, health, minds, and spirits," says medical intuitive Caroline Myss. "From an energy point of view, every choice that enhances our spirits strengthens our energy field; and the stronger our energy field, the fewer our connections to negative people and experiences."[21] For those of us on the quest to discover our best selves, who have committed to healing and our own inner work, and who have embraced being perfectly imperfect, shungite can help enhance our internal power—and resolve—to do what's best for us.

Everything is connected. What's in highest and best for us is also what's in highest and best for all those around us. Whether you're looking for something to help you manage how you're affected by the external world or looking to do

---

21 Caroline M. Myss, *Anatomy of the Spirit: The Seven Stages of Power and Healing* (New York: Three Rivers Press, 2004), 173.

some deep self-work, shungite can empower you to stay committed to your goals, stay grounded during moments of discomfort, and see the bigger picture in this thing called life.

With so many ways to use shungite to protect, manage, and enhance our energy, the effects it can have on your life are endless, should you choose to consciously work with this powerful mineral. So the only question left to ask is: What's stopping you?

Bibliography

Agarwal, Ashok, Aditi Mulgund, Alaa Hamada, and Michelle Chyatte. "A Unique View on Male Infertility around the Globe." *Reproductive Biology and Endocrinology*, April 26, 2015. https://doi.org/10.1186/s12958-015-0032-1.

Becker, Robert O., and Gary Selden. *The Body Electric: Electromagnetism and the Foundation of Life*. New York: William Morrow and Company, 1998.

Browne, Malcolm W. "Nature, It Turns Out, Made a Molecule Long before People Did." *New York Times*, July 10, 1992.

Campbell, Joseph. *The Hero with a Thousand Faces*. Novato, CA: New World Library, 2008.

Centers for Disease Control and Prevention. "Radiation Studies: Ionizing Radiation." December 7, 2015. https://www.cdc.gov/nceh/radiation/ionizing_radiation.html

Ducharme, Jamie. "A Lot of Americans Are More Anxious than They Were Last Year, a New Poll Says." *Time*, May 8, 2018. https://time.com/5269371/americans-anxiety-poll.

Eden, Donna, and David Feinstein. *Energy Medicine: Balancing Your Body's Energies for Optimal Health, Joy, and Vitality*. New York: Jeremy P. Tarcher, 2008.

Firstenberg, Arthur. *The Invisible Rainbow: A History of Electricity and Life*. White River Junction, VT: Chelsea Green Publishing, 2020.

Frawley, David. *Ayurvedic Healing: A Comprehensive Guide*. New Delhi, India: Motilal Banarsidass, 2012.

Frawley, David. *Yoga and Ayurveda: Self-Healing and Self-Realization.* New Delhi, India: Motilal Banarsidass, 2008.

Gerber, Richard. *Vibrational Medicine: New Choices for Healing Ourselves.* Rochester, VT: Bear & Company, 1996.

Gienger, Michael. *Crystal Power, Crystal Healing: The Complete Handbook.* London: Cassell, 2015.

Guhr, Andreas, and Jörg Nagler. *Crystal Power: Mythology and Power: The Mystery, Magic and Healing Properties of Crystals, Stones and Gems.* Findhorn, Scotland: Earthdancer, 2006.

Hall, Judy. *The Crystal Bible: A Definitive Guide to Crystals.* Cincinnati, OH: Walking Stick Press, 2003.

Harari, Yuval Noah. *Sapiens: A Brief History of Humankind.* New York: Harper Perennial, 2015.

Haumann, Thomas, Uwe Munzenberg, Wolfgang Maes, and Peter Sierck. "HF-Radiation Levels of GSM Cellular Phone Towers in Residential Areas." In *Biological Effects of EMFs: 2nd International Workshop (Rhodes, Greece, 7–11 October 2002)*; Proceedings, edited by P. Kostarakis, vol. 1, 327–333. Ioannina, Greece: University of Ioannina, 2002.

Hawkins, David R. *Power vs. Force: The Hidden Determinants of Human Behavior.* Carlsbad, CA: Hay House, 2014.

Hickson, Alice, and Lilly Blumenthal. "The Self Care Obsession." *Tufts Observer*, March 25, 2019.

Hunt, Valerie V. *Infinite Mind: Science of the Human Vibrations of Consciousness.* Malibu, CA: Malibu Publishing, 1996.

International Agency for Research on Cancer. "IARC Classifies Radiofrequency Electromagnetic Fields as Possibly Carcinogenic to Humans." May 31, 2011. https://www.iarc.fr/wp-content/uploads/2018/07/pr208_E.pdf.

Judith, Anodea. *Wheels of Life: A User's Guide to the Chakra System.* Woodbury, MN: Llewellyn Publications, 2018.

Kıvrak, Elfide Gizem, Kıymet Kübra Yurt, Arife Ahsen Kaplan, Işınsu Alkan, and Gamze Altun. "Effects of Electromagnetic Fields Exposure on the Antioxidant Defense System." *Journal of Microscopy and Ultrastructure* 5, no. 4 (2017): 167–176. https://www.ncbi.nlm.nih.gov/pmc/articles/PMC6025786/.

Klimova, Regina, Sergey Andreev, Ekaterina Momotyuk, Natalia Demidova, Natalia Fedorova, Yana Chernoryzh, Kirill Yurlov, et al. "Aqueous Fullerene C_{60} Solution Suppresses Herpes Simplex Virus and Cytomegalovirus Infections." *Fullerenes, Nanotubes and Carbon Nanostructures* 28, no. 6 (2020): 487–499. https://doi.org/10.1080/1536383X.2019.1706495.

Lad, Usha, and Vasant Lad. *Ayurvedic Cooking for Self-Healing.* Albuquerque, NM: The Ayurvedic Press, 2006.

Lang, Sidney B., Andrew A. Marino, Garry Berkovic, Marjorie Fowler, and Kenneth D. Abreo. "Piezoelectricity in the Human Pineal Gland." *Bioelectrochemistry and Bioenergetics* 41, no. 2 (1996): 191–195. https://www.sciencedirect.com/science/article/abs/pii/S0302459896051471.

Lear, Richard. "The Root Cause in the Dramatic Rise of Chronic Disease." Dramatic Rise in Chronic Disease Project, May 2016. https://www.researchgate.net/publication/303673576.

LeDoux, Joseph. *Anxious: Using the Brain to Understand and Treat Fear and Anxiety.* New York: Penguin Books, 2015.

Ma, Easter Joy Sajo, Cheol-Su Kim, Soo-Ki Kim, Kwang Yong Shim, Tae-Young Kang, and Kyu-Jae Lee. "Antioxidant and Anti-Inflammatory Effects of Shungite against Ultraviolet B Irradiation-Induced Skin Damage in Hairless Mice." *Oxidative Medicine and Cellular Longevity* (2017): 7340143. https://www.ncbi.nlm.nih.gov/pmc/articles/PMC5574306.

Martinez, Zachary S., Edison Castro, Chang-Soo Seong, Maira R. Cerón, Luis Echegoyen, and Manuel Llano. "Fullerene Derivatives Strongly Inhibit HIV-1 Replication by Affecting Virus Maturation without Impairing Protease Activity." *Antimicrobial Agents and Chemotherapy*

60, no. 10 (2016): 5731–5741. https://aac.asm.org/content/
60/10/5731.

Martino, Regina. *Shungite: Protection, Healing, and Detoxification.*
Rochester, VT: Healing Arts Press, 2014.

Matthews Ronald E. "Harold Burr's Biofields Measuring the
Electromagnetics of Life." *Bioelectromagnetic and Subtle Energy
Medicine* 18, no. 2 (2007): 55–61. https://journals.sfu.ca/seemj
/index.php/seemj/article/view/401.

Melezhik, V. A., A. E. Fallick, M. M. Filippov, and O. Larsen.
"Karelian Shungite—An Indication of 2.0-Ga-Old Metamorphosed
Oil-Shale and Generation of Petroleum: Geology, Lithology and
Geochemistry." *Earth-Science Reviews* 47, nos.1–2 (1999): 1–40.
https://www.sciencedirect.com/science/article/abs/pii/
S0012825299000276?via=ihub.

Mercola, Joseph. *EMF*d: 5G, Wi-Fi & Cell Phones: Hidden Harms and
How to Protect Yourself.* Carlsbad, CA: Hay House, 2020.

Moon, Hibiscus. *Crystal Grids: How and Why They Work: A Science-
Based, Yet Practical Guide.* Charleston, SC: CreateSpace Independent
Publishing Platform, 2011.

Myss, Caroline M. *Anatomy of the Spirit: The Seven Stages of Power
and Healing.* New York: Three Rivers Press, 2004.

National Cancer Institute. "Electromagnetic Fields and Cancer." Last
modified January 3, 2019. https://www.cancer.gov/about-cancer/
causes-prevention/risk/radiation/electromagnetic-fields-fact-sheet.

National Institute of Diabetes and Digestive Kidney Diseases."
Digestive Diseases Statistics for the United States." November 1, 2014.
https://www.niddk.nih.gov/health-information/health-statistics/
digestive-diseases.

National Research Council (US) Committee to Evaluate the U.S.
Navy's Extremely Low Frequency Communications System Ecological
Monitoring Program. "EMF Measurements, Exposure Criteria, and
Dosimetry." In *An Evaluation of the U.S. Navy's Extremely Low Frequency
Communications System Ecological Monitoring Program.* Washington

DC: National Academies Press, 1997. https://www.ncbi.nlm.nih.gov/books/NBK233160.

National Toxicology Program. "Cellphone Radio Frequency Radiation Studies." National Institute of Environmental Health Sciences. n.d. https://www.niehs.nih.gov/health/materials/cell_phone_radiofrequency_radiation_studies_508.pdf.

Pall, Martin L. "Wi-Fi Is an Important Threat to Human Health." *Environmental Research* 164 (July 2018): 405–416. https://www.sciencedirect.com/science/article/pii/S0013935118300355.

Peen, J. R. A. Schoevers, A. T. Beekman, and J. Dekker. "The Current Status of Urban-Rural Differences in Psychiatric Disorders." *Acta Psychiatrica Scandinavica* 121, no. 2 (2009): 84–93. https://pubmed.ncbi.nlm.nih.gov/19624573/.

Permutt, Philip. *The Complete Guide to Crystal Chakra Healing: Energy Medicine for Mind, Body, and Spirit.* London: CICO Books, 2009.

Pew Research Center. "Demographics of Mobile Device Ownership and Adoption in the United States." June 5, 2020. https://www.pewresearch.org/internet/factsheet/mobile.

Plante, Amber. "How the Human Body Uses Electricity." University of Maryland Graduate School. *The Grad Gazette*, February 2016. https://www.graduate.umaryland.edu/gsa/gazette/February-2016/How-the-human-body-uses-electricity/.

Schumann, Walter. *Gemstones of the World.* New York: Sterling, 2013.

Shoji, Masaki, Etsuhisa Takahashi, Dai Hatakeyama, Yuma Iwai, Yuka Morita, Riku Shirayama, Noriko Echigo, et al. "Anti-Influenza Activity of C_{60} Fullerene Derivatives." *PLoS One* 8, no. 6 (2013): e66337. https://www.ncbi.nlm.nih.gov/pmc/articles/PMC3681905.

Smith, Fritz Fredrick. *Inner Bridges: A Guide to Energy Movement and Body Structure.* Atlanta, GA: Humanics Publishing Group, 1998.

Sushko, V. O., O. O. Kolosynska, O. M. Tatarenko, G. A. Nezgovorova, Zh. M. Berestjana, S. I. Ustinov, and D. D. Hapeyenko. "Problems of Medical Expertise for Diseases that Bring to Disability and Death as a Result of Radiation Exposure Influence in Conditions of the

Chernobyl Catastrophe in Remote Postaccidental Period." *Problems of Radiation Medicine and Radiobiology* 23 (2018): 471–480. https://pubmed.ncbi.nlm.nih.gov/30582864.

Svoboda, Robert. *Ayurveda: Life, Health, and Longevity*. Albuquerque, NM: Ayurvedic Press, 2004.

University of Pennsylvania School of Medicine. "One in Four Americans Develop Insomnia Each Year: 75 Percent of Those with Insomnia Recover." *ScienceDaily*, June 5, 2018. https://www.sciencedaily.com/releases/2018/06/180605154114.htm.

Van der Kolk, Bessel A. *The Body Keeps the Score: Brain, Mind, and Body in the Healing of Trauma*. New York: Penguin Books, 2015.

Vandenbroucke, M., and C. Largeau. "Kerogen Origin, Evolution and Structure." *Organic Geochemistry* 38, no. 5 (2007): 719–833. https://www.sciencedirect.com/science/article/abs/pii/S014663800700006X.

Willard, Jill. *Intuitive Being: Connect with Spirit, Find Your Center, and Choose an Intentional Life*. New York: HarperOne, 2016.

Wilson, Sarah. *First, We Make the Beast Beautiful*. London: Corgi Books, 2019.

Zion, Tina M. *Reiki Teacher's Manual: A Guide for Teachers, Students, and Practitioners*. Atlanta, GA: Boutique of Quality Books, 2020.

Acknowledgments

This book would not have been possible without the support and help of some truly amazing people.

First, I'd like to thank the amazing team at Ulysses, who helped make this book a reality. Director of Editorial and Acquisitions Casie Vogel, thank you for taking a chance on me to get this book out into the world. Tyanni Niles, I am so grateful to have had you as my touchstone and liaison throughout this entire process. Thank you for your unending patience and understanding. Scott Calamar and Renee Rutledge, thank you for your eagle eyes and editorial prowess in helping to shape this into a truly amazing book about a truly amazing crystal.

I would like to thank my amazing friends Lindsay Tauscher and Cami Wolff for being my lending library for some of the books I referenced to make *Healing with Shungite* happen. Since this book was written entirely during the COVID-19 pandemic, I was unable to physically visit libraries in search of texts to support much of the data reported in this book. Your generosity in loaning me some of your gems during this time helped much of this book come together.

To my friends Suzanne Deisher, Cynthia Gamarra, Kaitlyn Leaf, and Micah Norgard: Thank you for your unending support and for being my rocks in times of uncertainty.

To my mother and sister: Thank you for your patience, support, and understanding during this strange yet exciting time. Thank you especially for allowing me to have a room of my own for writing and respite and for all the laughs and memories we made in the three months we spent together during this process.

I would also like to thank my students for being so understanding of my teaching sabbatical during this writing period to focus on the book. I am so grateful for your patience and support and hope that this book serves as a tool to help you manage in uncertain times.

This book would never have come to be had it not been for my chance encounter with the shungite crystal vendor I encountered in Miami at 2016's Seed Food & Wine week, who first introduced this powerful mineral to me. I am so grateful for the information you shared and for the first two pieces of shungite you sold me. Thank you isn't big enough.

Last but not least, this endeavor would not have been possible were it not for my partner, Brendan Bell. Thank you for holding my hand and my heart during this process, for believing in me when I found it hard to believe in myself. This book truly would never have come to be without you—and our sweet kitties—by my side. Thank you for the innumerable ways you supported me during this time—and all the ways you've always supported me. I love you.

About the Author

Jessica Mahler is a writer, Reiki master, breathwork facilitator, tarot reader, and yoga teacher based in Washington, DC. After the death of her best friend, she left her Brooklyn apartment and a successful career as a copy editor to live out of a suitcase in order to heal herself. Thanks to a series of serendipitous events and a surfboard, she learned about energy healing, uncovered a world filled with love and compassion, discovered her own magical gifts, and decided to dedicate her life to helping others find what she unearthed for herself. No matter the modality, Jessica aims to empower others to heal themselves by breaking free from their anxiety and limiting belief systems to connect to their own magic and potential to live a confident, more spiritually aligned life. Her writing has been featured in *Vogue*, *Bust*, *Laika*, *Men's Journal*, and *Shape*, among other outlets.